Psychiatry in General Practice

Part 1: Principles

DEDICATION

to my mother and father

Psychiatry in General Practice

Part 1: Principles

Edited by Ben Green

Lecturer in Psychological Medicine
Royal Liverpool University Hospital
University of Liverpool, UK

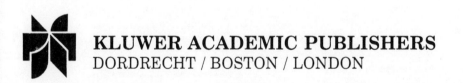

KLUWER ACADEMIC PUBLISHERS
DORDRECHT / BOSTON / LONDON

Also by Ben Green and published by Kluwer Academic Publishers:

MCQs for Finals, 1988, 90 pages, ISBN 0-7462-0102-8

More MCQs for Finals, 1990, 93 pages, ISBN 0-7923-8928-X

MCQs for MRCGP (edited by Ben Green), 1991, 94 pages,
ISBN 0-7923-8965-4

The MRCPsych Study Manual (edited by Ben Green), 1993,
160 pages, ISBN 0-7923-8816-X

Distributors

for the United States and Canada: Kluwer Academic Publishers, PO Box 358, Accord Station, Hingham, MA 02018-0358, USA

for all other countries: Kluwer Academic Publishers Group, Distribution Center, PO Box 322, 3300 AH Dordrecht, The Netherlands

A catalogue record for this book is available from the British Library.
ISBN 0-7923-8851-8

Published in the United Kingdom by Kluwer Academic Publishers, PO Box 55, Lancaster.

Kluwer Academic Publishers BV incorporates the publishing programmes of D. Reidel, Martinus Nijhoff, Dr W. Junk and MTP Press.

Printed and bound in Great Britain by Hartnolls Ltd., Bodmin, Cornwall.

Contents

Contributors

Dr Ben Green, MB, ChB, MRCPsych

Lecturer in Psychological Medicine, University Department of Psychiatry, Royal Liverpool University Hospital, PO Box 147, University of Liverpool, L69 3BX

Dr Chris Dowrick, BA, MB, ChB, MSc, CQSW, DRCOG, MRCGP

Senior Lecturer in General Practice, University Department of General Practice, PO Box 147, University of Liverpool, L69 3BX

Unattributed chapters are by the Editor.

Introduction

Psychiatry in General Practice is designed to meet the needs of the general practitioner – faced with a vast array of psychological distress and illness, but without lengthy psychiatric training, and the time resources used by psychiatrists. Part One looks at the symptoms and signs of mental disorder and how the current services operate to provide community care. Part Two looks at the problems faced by individuals and their families through their life cycles, together with a consideration of specific mental disorders, such as schizophrenia, and up-to-date management strategies.

Part One looks at the fundamental principles of psychopathology – the symptoms and signs of mental disorder and how to elicit them, confidently and quickly. The major advantage that psychiatrists have when interviewing their patients is time. The general practitioner has to use his or her time as effectively as possible, so that there is a real need to be as sensitive as possible to mental state abnormalities, such as low mood, and to be able to switch into specific question sets to crystallise diagnostic hypotheses as swiftly and as accurately as possible. The major advantages enjoyed by general practitioners in combatting mental illness are their community presence and knowledge of individuals and their families over time. Part One will enable the general practitioner to capitalise on these strengths. It includes:

- symptoms and signs of mental disorder, a glossary of terms and how to elicit features of the mental state precisely and confidently, screening questions for depression, schizophrenia and alcohol dependence
- a thumbnail classification of mental disorders ranging from dysthymia and anxiety to schizophrenia and organic disorders
- screening instruments for depression and dementia
- creating rapport, listening skills and counselling techniques
- the Mental Health Act and danger signals for violence and suicide
- current service organisation
- references and self-assessment exercises

Creating Rapport

In order to identify psychological distress and illness the doctor must create enough rapport with a patient to enable them to make their feelings known. Doctors use words and actions to create this rapport.

Different techniques are in use at different stages of the consultation. For the sake of convenience let us propose a simple five-stage model of a consultation:

- Introduction
- History and Clarification of Presenting Complaint
- Management Proposal
- Further Opportunity for Patient to Raise Concerns
- Close Down

1. Introduction

During this phase non-verbal behaviours play a key role in determining the acceptability of the doctor to the patient. The interview must be conducted in a comfortable, warm and private place, where the patient does not feel intimidated or as if he or she is about to be overheard or interrupted at any moment. If there is a difference between the seating of the doctor and the patient in terms of comfort or height, then this may accentuate alienation. The angle between the patient's and doctor's chairs should allow both individuals to regard one another without being so close or so opposite to one another as to suggest confrontation. Ideally there should be no desk to intrude upon or form a barrier to communication, but in practice a desk is essential to enable the doctor to write, or for the storage of stethoscopes, sphygmomanometers and other instruments. Given that we cannot dispense with the desk, then the seating should be carefully arranged around it and a portion of desk top space should be dedicated to the patient as his or her territory, to lean on or otherwise use.

Computers may save time, and may enhance efficiency, but the desktop terminal, keyboard and printer are much more intrusive than the notes and pen of yesteryear. Not only may the doctor appear preoccupied with a screen, but he or she may turn his head away from the patient to look at this screen. Patients are more susceptible to conscious and unconscious responses to such non-verbal behaviour than we think at first. Slow typing skills and an evident reliance on the pharmacological suggestions of the computer formulary do not enhance confidence.

Enhancing confidence is an important function of the introduction. Making direct eye contact, uttering an appropriate and tailored greeting, rising from the chair and perhaps shaking hands all communicate individual concern and care.

Summary of Communication Skills in Introductory Phase

Words	Actions
Greeting	Standing up
Use of Name	Making eye contact
Recognition Statements	Offering some physical contact
Orientation	e.g. handshake
e.g. "Hello, Mrs Carter. It's	Ensuring privacy
two months since I last saw you.	Positioning of chairs
I wanted to see you for a few	Showing patient to seat
minutes to ask you how things	Looking the part
were going with the	
counsellor"	

2. History and Clarification of Presenting Complaint

Open questions are most commonly used to explore the patient's agenda, unless the doctor pre-arranged the consultation, in which case he or she will need to start the agenda. To refresh your memory open questions are ones that can be answered in several ways of the patient's own choosing and effectively give control of the consultation to the patient. An example would be " How can I help you?" or "What would you like to talk about?" There are relatively few assumptions underlying such questions, except that the patient has come to the doctor for some reason, presumably to seek help. Closed questions make more assumptions, and require the doctor to have some hypothesis in mind which he or she wants to test out by seeking either a yes or no answer. Closed questions narrow down the field of answers that the patient can give. Examples of closed questions might be "Do you ever get chest pain?" or "Are you waking early in the morning?" Such closed questions may be *leading* – leading closed questions consciously or unconsciously force the patient into one particular answer. An example of a leading closed question might be: "You don't get worried about sex do you?" Doctors are often unaware that they use this kind of question. They are more likely to do so if it suits them to close down various fields of enquiry, for instance if they are uncomfortable talking about sex or pain.

Working from open to closed questions is sometimes referred to as coning. Closed questions are essential to clear up misunderstandings and to pursue diagnostic hypotheses. An interview therefore often proceeds in a series of cones, working from open to closed questions and back to open questions for the next section of enquiry.

Statements can be used in various ways. They can double as questions: "I'd like you to tell me about your family". They lead the patient to talk about certain things, but can also express empathy. The statement above begins "I'd like you to...", expressing an interest in the patient and their story. Statements can also be used to express concern more overtly. For instance after a patient has talked about a bereavement: "This must be very painful for you still". Such statements communicate understanding of the patient and their predicament. Psychiatrists often dissect out features of psycho-pathology without looking at the emotional reactions that psychotic symptoms provoke. The psychiatrist may be interested in determining whether an auditory hallucination is second person or third person, and may pursue the distinction without regard to the distress and fear that the patient feels because of the extraordinary experience they have had. Acknowledging the fear helps and a statement such as "That must have been frightening" may be sufficient to indicate concern, understanding and sympathy. Over-use of such statements may appear saccharin or insincere, and so their use should be carefully judged.

Statements can also be used to summarise the story so far. By such summaries the doctor conveys that they are attending and have understood. They also can give the patient an opportunity to correct any misconceptions on the part of the doctor. In psychotherapy statements are sometimes called *interpretations* – the psycho-therapist puts a hypothesis to the patient in the form of a statement and expects the patient to either accept or deny the interpretation; e.g. "It sounds like you and your Dad don't get on".

Non-verbal behaviours continue to be read by both patient and doctor throughout the interview. Videotapes of interviews can be startlingly revealing about body postures and pacing throughout the interview. Fleeting emotional responses, unseen during the interview can be identified when the interview is re-run.

Eye contact needs to be offered throughout the interview. Unflickering, continuous eye contact can be disturbing, so a balance is necessary. Patients who avoid eye contact may be anxious, depressed or deliberately evading issues.

Doctors often adopt similar bodily postures to their patients during the interview – leaning their elbows on the desk or putting their head on one side. In this way the doctor and patient can match or mirror each other. The exact meaning of such behaviour is open to interpretation, but if postures are linked and follow each other in a sequence (e.g. patient moves back in chair then doctor moves back in chair), it indicates an unconscious affinity, which may allow the patient to feel more relaxed and to unburden themselves. Discrepant postures may indicate a lack of rapport or anger on the part of doctor or patient.

A variety of noises can be used by the doctor to ease the conversation: grunts, uh-huhs, and similar meaningless noises that spur the patient on by indicating interest, but not much more. The doctor may be unaware of how little or how much he or she uses these. Over-use, particularly of idiosyncratic noises, can be distracting and irritating and may affect rapport adversely. For instance, if a doctor constantly repeats the meaningless phrase 'right-you-are' throughout the consultation, the patient can be frustrated by the habit. Again video or audio tapes can cruelly expose such behaviours, and the doctor may cringe at his or her own idiosyncrasies, but at least such tapes can make the doctor aware of these behaviours. Being aware of the problem can enable the doctor to change, reduce or vary the noises used in future interviews.

Pauses are often uncomfortable for new doctors. We can all remember the seemingly awkward silences as student doctors when we racked our brains trying to think of the next question to ask a patient. Pauses can be used after a patient has apparently stopped speaking. Prolonged silences can be uncomfortable, and so some people advocate that pauses should last between four and ten seconds. Advantages of such pauses are that they give the patient time to think about their next sentence and reflect on how the interview is going, they may also allow the disclosure of emotions, or something that the patient feels is sensitive information. Pauses humanise the conversation – a swift exchange of questions and answers can resemble nothing less than an interrogation. Long pauses can seem confrontational, but may be used, particularly in counselling situations when somebody is struggling with difficult memories or emotions, and wondering how they can put these into words.

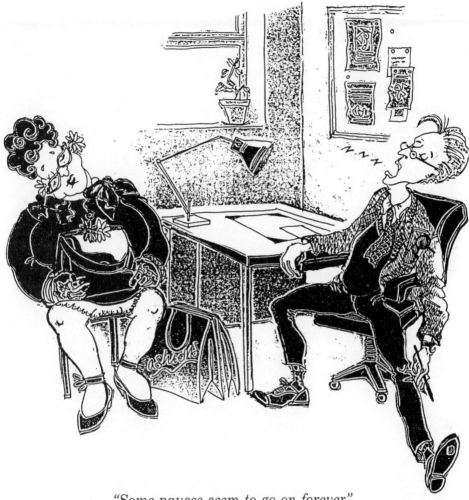

"Some pauses seem to go on forever"

3. Management Proposal

Assuming that a working or final diagnosis has been made, some management strategy will have emerged in the doctor's mind. Such a strategy may involve onward referral, investigations in the practice, temporising, or straightforward prescription. Whatever the management proposal is, it now needs to be conveyed, clearly and concisely.

Imparting bad news is never easy and never enjoyable. Parents of children with life-threatening illness interviewed by Wooley et al. (1989) had several wishes as to how bad news should be conveyed – including privacy, an uninterrupted and unhurried interview, often with a relative present, with due respect, use of names, with good eye contact, and direct, open, sympathetic communication. Rather than protecting people from bad news the information needs to be paced to what they are prepared to accept at any one time. The doctor needs to gauge the patient's or relative's readiness to ask or know more about the illness (Buckman, 1993). Emotions of self-blame, anger and defence mechanisms, particularly denial of the diagnosis, need to be borne in mind. Listen carefully to the concerns of the patient/relative – avoiding, where possible, the negative doctor-centred behaviours identified by Byrne and Long (1989).

Negative Doctor-Centred Behaviours (Byrne and Long, 1989)

- Rejecting patient offers
- Reinforcing self-position
- Denying patient
- Refusing patient ideas
- Evading patient questions
- Not listening
- Refusing to respond to feelings

There is often a temptation to reassure too early (mainly to alleviate the anxiety of the doctor rather than anything else). Reassurance is indeed comforting when appropriate, but reassurance before investigations are complete can be premature and ultimately prove false. However, hopeful aspects of treatment and prognosis should be realistically presented, to offset patient expectations that might be catastrophically negative.

During such difficult interviews, and also during less emotionally demanding interviews, it is difficult for both parties to recall exactly what has been said. The doctor should, as a matter of course, make notes of the main points, but writing things down for the patient or giving information sheets may be a valid additional behaviour. Explicit instructions for taking prescribed medications, or management plans may be essential to obtain compliance.

A further interview should be clearly offered, particularly where difficult issues have been discussed. Indeed, such an interview may be arranged there and then, and the patient encouraged to think about issues and write down matters that concern them for discussion in the next interview.

Doctors and patients may not always see eye-to-eye. Management proposals may not be acceptable to the patient – a doctor may feel it is

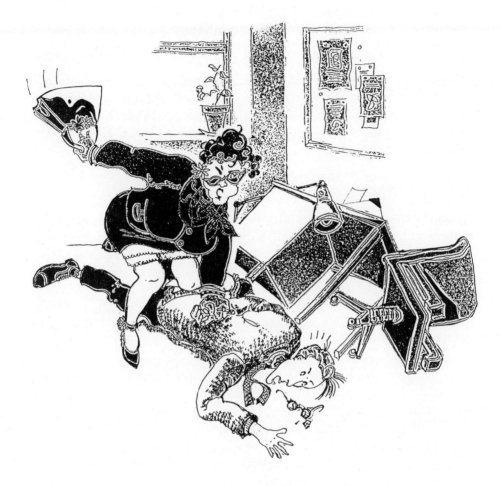

"Not always seeing eye-to-eye"

appropriate to refuse a repeat prescription for benzodiazepines, or may propose a referral for investigations that the patient dreads.

Under such circumstances it may be appropriate to maintain the management proposed (if it does seem correct), but the patient's point of view and emotional concerns need to be carefully explored. Reflecting back emotional responses can defuse difficult situations. Patients (and doctors) can seethe with rage at the actions of the other, while maintaining an icy politeness. Statements such as "You seem upset/anxious/angry/sad about that. I would like you to tell me why", may reveal surprising information (and sometimes enable clarification and resolution of differences), but reduce the likelihood of acting-out, particularly of violence.

4. Further Opportunity for Patient to Raise Concerns

When everything appears to have been settled, a further open question is necessary to elicit any further concerns. Such end-of-the-consultation concerns are often the main concern of the patient. Even if time is short such open questions need to appear to be unhurried, or the invitation will not be taken up.

5. Close Down

The interview close-down is often communicated by mutual exchange of non-verbal behaviours – e.g. the doctor sitting back in his/her chair, appearing to be about to get up, putting the notes away, or the patient gathering his/her things together, looking as if they are turning in their chair about to get up – and other signals.

A clear statement that the interview is at an end may be necessary with garrulous patients or potentially aggressive patients. Often such a statement seems less harsh if you have clearly defined how long the interview is to last at the outset.

Closing statements may include limited information such as advice to make a further appointment, or may re-orient the patient and doctor to an outside world (wishes for a Happy Christmas, or a comment about the patient's home life).

Final behaviours can include opening the door for the patient and a shake of the hand or a light squeeze of the upper arm, with an appropriate farewell.

Audit Points

- *Although we may consider our communication skills to be good, it is possible for our skills to 'drift' over time. Using a checklist of behaviours (as outlined overleaf) and checking these against videos or audio tapes of routine consultations, make a profile of your interviewing style. Using this profile, is there anything about your style which you would wish to change?*

- *Consider running an audit in the practice to ask patients what doctor behaviours they like during consultations, and in what ways doctors could make themselves easier to talk to. The audit might look at the whole interview or just at specific behaviour areas such as greetings, or the breaking of bad news. How would you run such an audit – by questionnaire or by structured interview?*

Self-Assessment

Before changing any aspect of our consultation skills we need first to be aware of our normal behaviour. Setting up video or audio taping equipment can be useful to monitor our interactions with patients*. Naturally such tapes have to be made with patient consent, and the aim of such tapes has to be fully explained to the patient. Role-playing can sometimes be used as an alternative. In role playing it is useful to have three people, one to be the patient, one to be the doctor, and one to be the monitor who scores the behaviour checklist (Green et al., 1991).

Using the following checklist you can produce a profile of the consultation. Doctors can see from the profile how often they use various behaviours. They may note that they rarely use statements or over-use reassurance. They will be able to see their strengths and areas where they can make changes. Hopefully such conscious changes will improve the quality of consultations.

* Checklists for audiotaped interview behaviour can be found in Byrne and Long (1989) and in Lieberman and Cobb (1987).

Video Checklist

Non-verbal behaviours	Frequency or presence
Welcoming gesture (e.g. standing up/shaking hands)	
Appropriate eye contact	
Congruent posture	
Patient-orientated seating	
Attending primarily to patient (not notes or computer)	
Nodding or facilitatory gestures	
Verbal behaviours	
Pauses	
Encouraging noises	
Use of patient's name	
Open question	
Closed question	
Leading closed question	
Open to closed question structure	
Introductory statement	
Reassuring statement	
Summarising statement	
Prescribing statement (giving new information)	
Checking/clarifying statement	
Self-disclosing statement	
Empathic statement	
Reflecting patient's emotion	

References and Further Reading

Balint, M. (1964) The Doctor, his Patient and the Illness. London, Pitman.

Balint, M, Balint, E. (1961) The doctor's emotions. Chapter in: Psychotherapeutic Techniques in Medicine. Tavistock, London.

Bennet, G. (1987) The Wound and the Doctor. Healing, Technology and Power in Modern Medicine. Secker and Warburg, London.

Book, H E. (1988) Empathy – misconceptions and misuse in psychotherapy. American Journal of Psychotherapy, 145, 420–424.

Buckman, R. (1993) How to Break Bad News. London, Macmillan.

Byrne, P S, Long, B E L. (1989) Doctors Talking to Patients. London, Royal College of General Practitioners.

Green, B H , Göpfert, M, Dickinson, P, Abou-Saleh, M. (1991) Developing therapeutic interview skills in medical students. Psychiatric Bulletin, 15, 157–158.

Leff, J P, Isaacs, A D. (1992) Difficult patients. Chapter in: Psychiatric Examination in Clinical Practice. Third Edition. London, Blackwell.

Lieberman, S, Cobb, J P. (1987) The grammar of psychotherapy. Interactograms: three self-monitoring instruments for audiotape feedback. British Journal of Psychiatry, 151, 594–601.

Nuffield working party on communications with patients. (1980) Talking with Patients. A Teaching Approach. London, Nuffield Hospitals Provincial Trust.

Royal College of General Practitioners. (1972) The Future General Practitioner. Learning and Teaching. London, British Medical Journal.

Woolley, H, Stein, A, Forrest, G C, Baum, J D. (1989) Imparting the diagnosis of life threatening illness in children. British Medical Journal, 298, 1623–1626.

Symptoms and Signs of Mental Disorder

Objectives

To refresh basic aspects of psychiatry. After working through this chapter you should be familiar again with:

- the main symptoms and signs of mental illness
- how to take a full psychiatric history
- how to perform a mental state examination
- the new main diagnostic classification of mental illness (ICD-10)
- how to summarise a patient's history and work out a differential diagnosis

Introduction

- Psychiatrists use four methods of assessment: the psychiatric history, a mental state examination, a physical examination and relevant medical, social and psychological investigations.

- Information from these assessment methods is built into a differential diagnosis, from which a management plan is formulated. The assessment is a holistic one in that it incorporates physical, social and psychological components. Similarly treatments for mental illness may involve physical, social and psychological treatments.

- Physical treatments may include drugs such as antidepressants and antipsychotics, electroconvulsive therapy (ECT) and, very rarely, psychosurgery.

- Social treatments may involve re-housing in special rehabilitation settings, attendance at day hospital or day centres, some family interventions such as giving information and counselling to relatives, and socio-legal advice.

- Psychological treatments may include one-to-one psychotherapy, group psychotherapy, and family therapy. One-to-one psychotherapy is sometimes called interpersonal therapy. There are many different forms such as psychoanalysis and cognitive therapy.

- However, such treatment plans can only be put into place, once a diagnosis is made, and before a doctor can make a diagnosis, he or she must first recognise the symptoms and signs of mental illness. Such symptoms and signs are referred to as *psychopathology*.

Psychopathology

Throughout life we experience a variety or spectrum of emotions and thoughts. Only when these emotions or thoughts become excessively severe, persistent or dominant do they become pathological. For instance, it is a normal reaction to feel sadness after a bereavement or some other set-back in life, such as failing to get or losing a job. If that sadness becomes unduly persistent, or so severe that it dominates an individual's life, (e.g., affecting their sleep or their appetite and leading to ideas of suicide) then it assumes a pathological character and becomes a depressive illness.

Abnormal Moods

Emotions can be fleeting, but emotional tones may persist for hours or days when they might better be termed moods or affects. Pathological mood states are called affective disorders.

Excessively severe or persistent sadness may be termed *depression*. Depression is associated with tearfulness or feeling that one is on the edge of tears. Sometimes in severe depression the sufferer may say that they feel they have 'gone beyond crying'. Depressed people have a negative view of themselves, the world in general and the future. They may feel there is no point in carrying on and may minimise their own worth. This feeling of worthlessness may be aggravated by a feeling of guilt and sufferers may ruminate on past actions that they now regret. Depressed people become underactive and may feel their thoughts are slowed down. To people watching them they may actually seem slowed down, perhaps sitting motionless in a chair for hours on end, or taking to their beds. There are alterations in sleep, eating, sexual and bowel habits. The so-called biological features of depression include:

- Poor sleep with initial insomnia (difficulty getting off to sleep), wakefulness, and early morning wakening (waking much earlier than usual and unable to get back to sleep).

- Poor appetite (fewer meals and less eaten) – depressed people complain that food is tasteless and that they are not hungry, similarly, depressed people may stop drinking too.
- Weight loss (depressed people may starve themselves to death).
- Decreased libido (depressed people are generally less interested in sex).
- Constipation.
- Diurnal mood variation (feeling more depressed in the morning).

Mild and moderate depression may include variants of the above, but severe depression may include additional *psychotic* features, such as auditory hallucinations and delusions. The psychotic features fit closely with the depressed mood so that if the patient generally feels worthless auditory hallucinations will reinforce this – so the person may hear voices telling them they are worthless, or evil. Delusions will fit in with the depressed mood too, so the depressed person may have delusions that they are evil and have committed some horrendous crime and have to be punished. Delusions of ill-health (hypochondriacal delusions), or infestation, or poverty may also occur. A severe form of delusion in depression is a nihilistic delusion, e.g that they have no bowels in their abdomen, or no brains in their head.

Such psychotic symptoms are rare in depression. Milder forms of depression may affect 10–18% of the population.

The extreme opposite of depression is *mania*. A manic affect is characterised by extreme happiness (elation or euphoria). Whereas in depression thoughts and actions are often slowed down, in mania thoughts seem to race and the sufferer may be overactive. There is a feeling of great well-being and the patient may feel they are invincible or very rich. Unlike the depressive ideas of worthlessness, the manic person may feel they have special powers or talents or even have a grandiose delusion such that, say, they can save the world. The manic person may not feel the need to sleep and may work all night long, they may over-eat, exercise excessively and be sexually promiscuous. They may make bad decisions and spend excessively. Since they feel so well, they may deny that they are unwell (*poor insight*). A lesser form of mania, *hypomania*, is more common. Irritability may accompany mania, and because of disinhibition such irritable manic patients may be violent.

In chronic psychiatric illnesses such as schizophrenia the affect may become restricted (blunted affect), the subject reports that his emotions are never stimulated to joy or sadness, and to the observer the individual with blunted affect seems less than animated in conversation.

Abnormal Thoughts

Psychiatrists are interested in thought in terms of its *form* and its *content*. Abnormalities in terms of form may be perceived as a disturbance in the stream of thought. Abnormalities may be recognised as breaks in the stream of thought, (such as thought blocking), slowing down of the stream of thought (as in psychomotor retardation in depression), racing thoughts (recognised by pressure of speech or flight of ideas), or a complete breakdown of the logical flow of thought (as in thought disorder, where the associations between thoughts become distorted). Thought blocking is characteristic of schizophrenia, and is a distressing phenomenon where a thought is abruptly lost. In pressure of speech words are uttered very rapidly, indicating a rapid progression of thought. In flight of ideas, the speech is usually pressured and ideas which are flowing equally quickly are often only linked by verbal puns or like-sounding words, (e.g. rhymes or clang associations). The key thing is that there is an association between the ideas, e.g.

"I'm wearing sandals, third world shoes, road to Damascus shoes, conversions shoes, converting light into spirit, whisky makes you frisky, gin makes you sin, bright as a pin, light as a kite."

In thought disorder (usually seen in schizophrenia) this association between ideas is lost or at least very obscure (sometimes called loosening of associations, knight's move thinking, or derailment). Terms for severe thought disorder (where very few words or phrases are understandable) include word salad and schizophasia. Words in thought disordered patients may be misused or invented (these new words are called neologisms).

"I Arthur Smith do hereby invest the albigeration of alogistical neophancy with the purple stream of rushing personae, amplified by the univariate clouds of forgiven angels, dancing in the sodden sun."

Apart from the form that thoughts take, abnormalities may also occur in terms of the content of that thought. We all have worries from time to time, but when these dominate our waking hours they may be termed *preoccupations*. Mildly depressed patients may be preoccupied with regrets about their childhood and things they have done wrong in the past.

When unwelcome or absurd thoughts repeatedly enter the mind (such as a recurrent urge to wash one's hands or to perform some ritual such as touching light switches eight times before switching them on) and are recognised as absurd by the individual, these may be termed intrusive thoughts and are suggestive of obsessive–compulsive disorder.

Occasionally people develop systematised ideas on obscure themes such as Unidentified Flying Objects; where these dominate their lives to some extent, but are nevertheless on the edges of cultural beliefs and are not held with rigid conviction (so that in an argument the individual might concede that their ideas may possibly be wrong, but still hold on to them), these may be termed over-valued ideas. There is an almost complete spectrum of pathological ideas ranging away from normal towards increasingly abnormal forms, e.g. firstly preoccupations, then onwards to intrusive thoughts, to over-valued ideas and finally to delusions.

When an individual holds beliefs which are absurd, or wrong and which are beyond culturally accepted norms (e.g. a belief that God lives in their toilet cistern) and held by that person with a rigid unshakeable conviction, these are delusions. Primary delusions occur *de novo*, i.e. without a precipitant, and are sometimes called *autochthonous delusions*. Secondary delusions occur as by-products of an abnormal experience such as hallucinations or abnormal affect. An example may be a delusion that one is the son of the devil after being told this by 'the voice of God'. Delusions are characteristic of psychotic illness. Different kinds of delusions may occur.

- Persecutory delusions may occur in severe depressive disorders and paranoid schizophrenia. In this type of delusion the individual feels under threat by some external agency, for instance the CIA, the Freemasons or the police, and believe they are under surveillance, or being poisoned.

- Grandiose delusions may occur in schizophrenia and hypomania. In these a person overestimates their powers, resources or abilities. A patient may believe they are a gifted pop star (when in fact they cannot play a note) or a Government Minister, an angel or even God.

- Delusions of guilt are often a feature of depressive disorder and are congruent with the low mood and poor self-esteem. An example of a delusion of guilt might be a certain knowledge that one is personally and wholly responsible for famine in the Third World.

- Delusions of reference occur when normal unrelated events seem especially contrived or have a special meaning for the individual, e.g the radio playing a song by Elton John entitled "You're my baby" means that their infant son is Elton John's child.

- Delusions of ill-health may occur in severe depressive illness: someone of thirty-five may believe they are riddled with cancer (when they are not). Delusions of infestation *(Ekbom's syndrome)* may also occur; e.g. that one's skull is filled with cockroach eggs, or one's stomach is filled with worms. Nihilistic delusions are a feature of severe depressive illness and may take the form of believing that one has no bowels *(Cotard's syndrome)*, or no brains, or that time does not exist beyond tomorrow.

- Delusional perception occurs when a normal perception is suddenly heavily invested with meaning and immediately associated with delusional significance e.g. "when I saw the sun come out from behind the clouds I knew for certain that I was going to give birth to the new Messiah".

Abnormal Experiences

In altered states of consciousness, extremes of mood, during and after epileptic attacks, and in mental illness, normal sensory perceptions may be distorted or abnormally generated. In *micropsia* visual perceptions appear abnormally small. In *macropsia* visual perceptions appear over-large. In *xanthopsia* visual perceptions are coloured yellow. In *hyperacusis* normal sounds appear over-loud. Normal perceptions can be altered at a cortical level through extremes of mood or affect or altered levels of consciousness. Fear produces an increased level of arousal, and normal sensory images may be altered by the cortex into frightening images which are examples of *illusions*. Illusions are sensory deceptions. In an illusion an actual perception is altered in some way, so that a stain on the wallpaper might appear as a wolf's head. However, if a sensory perception is not triggered by some external reality, for instance if someone saw a wolf's head with no external stimulus (such as the wallpaper stain), this would be termed an *hallucination*. Illusions and hallucination can occur in any sensory modality. Hallucinations, then, are abnormal sensory perceptions that are experienced as if they were real, in external space, and without an original or direct stimulus from the environment.

A patient's affect may determine the kind of hallucination they have. In depression any auditory hallucinations (voices) may be threatening or accusatory. The hallucinations may then form the origin of a false belief. Secondary persecutory delusions (such as "the Freemasons are out to get me. They wait outside my house 24 hours a day") may have its origin in an hallucination where the individual hears the voice of the devil telling him he has been bad and will be kept under surveillance by the Freemasons. In this case the delusion is secondary to the hallucination.

Hallucinations most commonly take auditory forms: visual hallucinations are less common and sometimes have an organic basis. Somatic, gustatory and olfactory hallucinations are those of touch, taste and smell respectively. Olfactory hallucinations may occur in severe depressive disorders ("I can smell my own rotting flesh") or in organic brain lesions, e.g. those affecting the frontal lobe. Hallucinations usually indicate severe or psychotic mental illness. However, when people are falling asleep or waking they may have what are termed *hypnagogic* or *hypnopompic* hallucinations. These occur occasionally in most people, whether or not they are mentally ill. Another occasion when 'normal' people might have a hallucinatory-like experience is following a bereavement when they might hear or see the recently-dead. This *pseudohallucination of mourning* is driven by an innate wish to see the dead one, and arises as a function of expectancy more than anything. Such pseudohallucinations are typically very brief and are not taken to be reality by the individual.

True hallucinatory voices making accusations or derogatory comments in depression are often addressed to the patient and are known as *second person auditory hallucinations*. Second person auditory hallucinations are voices talking *to* the patient. In schizophrenia voices may comment on the patient in conversation with other voices, (e.g. in a running commentary: "he's moving about the room now" or "she's reading her psychiatry book now"). In addition the voices may converse about thoughts or feelings that the patient may have. Voices talking about the patient are known as *third person auditory hallucinations*.

Patients with schizophrenia sometimes hear their thoughts spoken aloud as they think them (*gedankenlautwerden*) or echoed by a voice (*thought echo*).

Abnormal experiences may include alterations of the experience of self. When people are tired or unwell they may have the experience of *depersonalisation* – when they feel unreal, or apart from the world. This may occur in 'normal' people when they are abnormally stressed, or as an epileptic aura, or in any mental illness. Depersonalisation is therefore not particularly characteristic of any diagnosis. *Derealisation* is a variant of depersonalisation when the world around the person feels unreal. Abnormal experiences of time may occur as in *deja vu* and *jamais vu* (see glossary) – these again may be normal or neurotic symptoms, or may be a feature of temporal lobe epilepsy.

Psychotic experiences also include thought interference. This is more characteristic of schizophrenia than anything else, and occurs in various forms. In *thought insertion* the individual feels that thoughts are inserted into his mind. The thoughts therefore are not experienced as his or her own – they are alien thoughts. This distressing experience may be rationalised by the individual using a delusion – e.g. "John Major is putting thoughts into my head using a phrenological thought transmitter". In this case the delusion is secondary to the psychotic experience of thought insertion. *Thought withdrawal* is where the person feels that their thoughts are being removed from their mind by an external agency. *Thought broadcasting* is where the person feels their thoughts being transmitted from their mind, so that everyone knows their innermost thoughts. It is not 'as if' these things were happening to them, they actually experience these things happening to them.

A final variant of psychotic experience is the *passivity phenomenon*. In passivity phenomena the person feels that they are being controlled in some way by another agency. Their sovereignty over their own thoughts, feelings and actions has gone or been altered. Thought interference is sometimes classified as the thought equivalent of a passivity phenomenon. Classical passivity phenomena are made actions and made feelings. In made actions it feels to the person that, say, a movement of their leg or arm is being controlled by someone else. Similarly in made emotions their feelings are in some way controlled by another, e.g. "I am sad, but it is someone else's sadness" or "someone has been in my brain and taken the sincerity out of my emotion, it has been washed away". Typically, passivity phenomena are seen in schizophrenia.

The Psychiatric Assessment

There are four components to a psychiatric assessment:

- History
- Mental State Examination
- Physical Examination
- Investigations

The psychiatric history is lengthier and more detailed than in other fields of medicine. It seeks to cover aspects of personality, psychiatric illness and personal biography as well as a detailed medical history. To obtain this information the psychiatrist may interview the patient and an informant such as a relative, friend or other close acquaintance, (but only with the patient's consent). It is unlikely that a general practitioner will be able to invest the time necessary to take a full psychiatric history, although many general practitioners are very adept at the skill of finding the most important facts in the patient's life in a very short time indeed. The following section covers the questions that psychiatrists feel are important in their initial assessment interview and which might be used by general practitioners when they feel these are appropriate.

Since the history seeks to include sensitive information about past events and about feelings past and present, it is important to remember that patients need time, and need to feel that their doctor is genuinely interested if they are to disclose personal details. Accordingly psychiatric interviews are less controlled by the doctor and involve the use of more open questions and empathic statements by the doctor. Open questions are often used at the beginning of a section of questions, say, on family history and will allow the patient to talk about important aspects as they see them, e.g. "Can you begin by telling me about your family?" Even so, to regain control of the interview or gather specific information closed questions will still need to be used, e.g. "What age was your father when he died?" or "Which drugs helped you in the past?" or "Do you ever feel like harming yourself?"

Statements, if used carefully, can show that you understand what the patient is talking about from their point of view. Psychotic experiences are distressing ones, associated with fear. Acknowledging this in some way can make a patient think that their doctor knows something about the symptoms, but also understands how they really feel. Being understood is a positive experience for the patient and is reassuring.

After a suitable introduction, a psychiatrist would take down the patient's demographic details, including the patient's age, marital status, employment status and, if in hospital, whether they are there voluntarily or are on a section of the 1983 Mental Health Act (i.e. are compulsorily detained). Patient's ages, marital and employment status all have a bearing on their diagnosis and management. Different mental illnesses come on at different ages. Schizophrenia has its main onset in the third decade, dementia in the seventh and subsequent decades. The unemployed are more likely to suffer from depression, and suicides are more common in the unmarried, widowed and divorced.

The presenting complaint is usually a brief list of the major problems as seen by the patient e.g. 'hearing voices in the loft' or 'drinking too much alcohol'. The History of Presenting Complaint (HPC) records further details. In terms of details it is sometimes useful to compare psychological pain, e.g. depression, with physical pain. Surgeons will inquire as to the severity of the pain, its character, its onset, whether it is persistent or not and whether it is getting better or is aggravated by any particular thing. Similarly in a case of depression psychiatrists are interested in how it started: Did it start suddenly or gradually? Did anything happen to bring on the depression such as a bereavement or a loss of job, or was the onset insidious and gradual? Similarly, is the pain getting worse or better? Can it be made better by visitors or entertainment or is it persistent? Psychiatrists also ask for biological features of depression such as poor sleep, (particularly early morning wakening), poor appetite (or anorexia), weight loss (secondary to anorexia), diurnal mood variation, psychomotor retardation, loss of sexual energy and impulses, and constipation. The HPC would also focus on how severe the depression felt – is the patient crying every day or only once a week? It is sometimes appropriate to ask at this point whether the patient feels that life is worth living, and if not, then has the depressed patent thought about harming themselves and do they have any definite plans? Similarly if a patient complained of hearing voices an attempt would be made to discern exactly what these voices were like – were they hallucinations or illusions, for instance. If the doctor suspected schizophrenia it would be appropriate in the HPC to ask for other features of schizophrenia, just as in a case of suspected appendicitis the surgeon would ask about fever and features of urinary tract infection to aid in making his or her differential diagnosis.

In the past psychiatric history the doctor is trying to build up a picture of how the illness has affected the patient in the past. The psychiatrist wishes to know the onset of the illness and how many episodes there have been, who treated these illnesses and how successful they were – in particular which treatments were most useful. A useful probe at the beginning of this section might be "Have you ever felt like this before?" or "Have you ever seen a psychiatrist before?" Bear in mind though that not all psychiatric illness presents to psychiatrists or even to doctors at all, so that the true onset of an illness may be a long time before the psychiatrist is called in. Try and get a picture of how many episodes of illness there have been. How long did each episode last? And between episodes how well was the patient? Were they able to resume their work, or care for their family as usual?

Some illnesses impair function even between acute episodes. For any previous hospital admission you need to know which hospital it was (useful for getting past notes), which consultant, how long the admission was for, and whether they were formally detained or were informal (voluntary). Record any use of antipsychotics, anti-depressants, benzodiazepines and electroconvulsive therapy (ECT).

The past medical history is particularly relevant. Psychological reactions can occur secondary to being ill. About 25% of medical in-patients have appreciable levels of depressive symptoms. In addition, physical illness may mimic mental illness (hypothyroidism may present with depression; serum B_{12} deficiency may present with dementia, hyperthyroidism may present with persecutory ideas; Cushing's syndrome may present with psychosis as may Huntington's disease and temporal lobe epilepsy; drugs that are used to treat physical illnesses may cause psychiatric presentations; cimetidine may cause confusion, propranolol may cause depression). Besides these areas of relevance psychological disturbance may be related to physical presentations (e.g. low back pain, headaches and other illnesses). Psychological conflicts may be somatised in this way. The psychiatrist is therefore interested in current and past physical problems including major operations (e.g. orchidectomy and hysterectomy may be complicated by depression and low esteem), head trauma (which may provoke epileptic phenomena) and medications.

Components of the Psychiatric History

History Items in Order	Brief Description
Demographic	Age/Marital and work status/Inpatient or outpatient/Mental Health Act status
Presenting Complaint and History of Presenting Complaint	List of main problems with details of how long these have lasted, how they started and whether they are getting better or worse. May include exploration of symptoms e.g. suicidal ideas.
Past Psychiatric History	First contact with psychiatry or onset of psychiatric illness, subsequent episodes, hospital admissions and treatments, previous uses of Mental Health Act.
Past Medical History	
Family History	Family tree with details of any psychiatric illnesses, relationships within the family, and physical illness. Probe for depression and suicide.
Personal History	Chronological biography from birth onwards, including school, work and loving relationships. Include forensic probes.
Social History	Current accommodation and co-habitees, any financial problems, smoking, alcohol, and illicit drug use history.
Drug History	Prescribed drugs in current use, previously used drugs if relevant, with dosages, for depots and all oral medication. Adverse drug reactions.
Premorbid Personality	Self-assessment of personality traits prior to the onset of any psychiatric illness.
Corroborative History	Additional information regarding symptoms and signs, compliance with treatment, drug, alcohol and forensic history where appropriate.

The family history should include details of parents, siblings and sometimes children. A brief probe should be made about mental illness and suicide in any other relatives. It sometimes helps to record the family history in family tree form with notes against each family member (see example overleaf). You should not be purely interested in the psychiatric history of other family members (although it is very relevant because certain psychiatric illnesses cluster in families). This is an opportunity to discuss the patient's feelings about parents and brothers and sisters (siblings). It is of great value to know, for instance, that a patient has never felt able to burden their mother with their anxieties, because the mother had suffered with depression as well, or that the father was an argumentative man with an alcohol problem

Family tree of a patient with depression

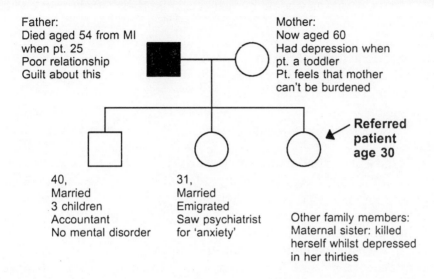

Father:
Died aged 54 from MI
when pt. 25
Poor relationship
Guilt about this

Mother:
Now aged 60
Had depression when
pt. a toddler
Pt. feels that mother
can't be burdened

Referred
patient
age 30

40,
Married
3 children
Accountant
No mental disorder

31,
Married
Emigrated
Saw psychiatrist
for 'anxiety'

Other family members:
Maternal sister: killed
herself whilst depressed
in her thirties

who used to beat his wife (the patient's mother). The family has been found to be important in the aetiology of personality difficulties, anorexia nervosa, bulimia nervosa and the prognosis of schizophrenia. Patients with schizophrenia are more likely to relapse in families where there is a high level of expressed emotion (hostility, over-involvement by other members, and high levels of face-to-face contact).

The personal history seeks to build up a biography from birth to the present day. Early events in a person's life can fundamentally change the course their life takes. Early separation can colour just how secure people are in all their subsequent relationships. Early perinatal brain damage can affect IQ, or lead to disabling epilepsy. There are hypotheses linking perinatal damage, febrile convulsions and adult psychotic illnesses. It is therefore important to know details as far back as possible. Gather information about the individual's birth – was it a normal full-term vaginal delivery, or an induced or instrumental birth? Was there any event, such as time spent in a special care baby unit that might have affected the maternal–infant relationship (perhaps making it a distant one, or even over-close)? Is there any evidence for delay in reaching milestones such as the first steps, or the first words? Can the person remember any details of what life was like when they were small. Were they hospitalised for any reason? Were they happy memories or not? Did they get on with their siblings? Can they remember what it was like when they first went to school? Did they mix easily and find happiness with plenty of friends or were they lonely individuals, constantly being bullied? How did their parents get along? Were there numerous rows, or was their home one filled with mutual affection? If there were rows, did the child feel responsible for them in any way? Sometimes children feel that they cause marital breakdowns, especially if these occur at the 'age of magical thinking' – when everything that happens in the outside world can be seen as a consequence of personal action; examples of magical thinking include "if I don't step on the lines in the pavement Mum and Dad will stay together'.

How did the person find the work at school...was it easy or was it very difficult for them? Were there any difficulties with reading delay or illiteracy? Were there any 'neurotic traits' such as prolonged bedwetting not due to organic causes, nailbiting, hair pulling, head-banging, or encopresis?

When the time came to move from primary to secondary education, how was that transition? Was it a smooth and easy one or was it fraught with anxiety? Was any time taken off school for exaggerated illness, (school refusal) or was there any truancy (with others or alone)? Did the person make new friends after the move? What were their favourite subjects at school? Any hobbies?

What qualifications or examinations did the person gain by the time they left school? This may give an indication of their intelligence level. What did they do after they left school? Put together a work history of where people worked and what they did, and for how long. If they left a job why did they leave? Was it because they were made redundant, got bored, found a better post, or were fired because they were difficult personalities, or because they were becoming mentally ill? In the early phases of illness people often underperform at work, especially when they suffer from depression and schizophrenia. Because of their low self-esteem, the depressed individual may think that their sacking is entirely justified and make no protest when in fact they were and are ill.

There are aspects of our lives which we usually keep to ourselves unless we are prompted to talk about them. This may be because they are potentially embarrassing or are aspects which will damage the way they are seen by others, such as impotence. Another person may not disclose his conviction for fraud because it will colour what you think of him. One of the barriers to disclosure is if the patient feels that their doctor is easily embarrassed or does not wish to discuss sensitive aspects of their lives. Unfortunately such sensitive aspects of people's lives are often the ones that cause them the most anxiety. Such patients suffer in silence. The doctor who shows a willingness to discuss such matters openly helps his or her patients disclose. Such aspects are often crucial to diagnosis and management and must not be ignored. No doubt when you were a student doctor you felt embarrassed in such discussions, but with experience in consultations over the years your discomfort has eased. Two such areas that you will need to cover in the personal history are the patient's psychosexual history and their forensic history (or criminal record).

What relevance is a patient's sexual history? It is important to realise that sexuality is inherent in all people regardless of their age, physical wellbeing or mental condition and is a major factor in their lives. Psychosexual functioning seems to have some bearing on prognosis. Good function suggests a reasonable premorbid personality and this correlates with a better prognosis. Sexual orientation is a problem for some people and this may provide a focus for psychotherapeutic interventions. Psychosexual function is also of value in making judgements about dangerousness in some sexual offenders. Doctors should therefore be interested in what kind of relationships the person builds up. *Schizoid personalities* tend to avoid contact with other people, especially sexual relationships, so their psychosexual history may be characterised by a complete absence or avoidance of sexuality. Their sexuality may though be expressed in isolation, by fantasy or masturbation. *Borderline personalities* sometimes have many intense, but fleeting sexual relationships. The relationships may be affected by discord or violence. In depressive illness there is often a reduced sexual drive, and this may cause difficulties with the partner. Similarly mania may lead to a heightening of sexuality, and a lack of judgment may put patients at risk because they have unprotected sex with people that they might not normally approach. Although a psychiatrist might have a duty to protect patients in such circumstances it is important to realise that sexuality itself, in the absence of mental disorder, is not a reason for the use of the Mental Health Act. At different times and places in history homosexuality and other sexual behaviours have been thought abnormal, or expressions of illness and therefore the province of doctors, and even the subject of compulsory detention orders. This is not the case today.

What features are included in the psychosexual history? We wish to know generally about the patient's current and past loving relationships. Are they a source of general pleasure and satisfaction or are they characterised by rows or unhappiness? Specifically we need to know when the person began building relationships – at what age?

What was their source of sexual education? What were their feelings about sex? How long did their first relationships last? Were they happy experiences or were there problems? How did they manage those problems? When was the first experience of sexual intercourse? Are the relationships heterosexual or homosexual? You need to know whether sex is pleasurable, merely satisfactory or if there are any specific sexual dysfunctions such as impotence, vaginismus or premature ejaculation.

A history of childhood sexual abuse may affect an individual's capacity to enjoy subsequent sexual relationships and may also have relevance to abnormal personality development, alcoholism, eating disorders and depression. Some psychiatrists include a screening question for sexual abuse in all their initial interviews (such as "These days more people seem able to talk about difficult things which have happened in their childhood. Some people are able to talk about how they were beaten as a child, or how sometimes older people took advantage of them sexually. Has anything like that ever happened to you?"). Other psychiatrists prefer to allow their patients to disclose at their own pace, although they create an atmosphere of trust and safety where the person can disclose what they wish when they wish. For some people disclosing past abuse is relatively easy, for others the disclosure and the fear of subsequent rejection by the doctor may make disclosure very threatening. Disclosures of ongoing abuse or violence, or disclosure that a minor is at risk, may necessitate immediate action to protect the individual or a third party.

A forensic history concerns the overlap between criminal offending behaviour and psychiatry. Patients with schizophrenia may harm others in response to second person auditory hallucinations telling them to do so. Many crimes may be committed by patients with drug or alcohol problems and these may be referred to specialist psychiatrists called forensic psychiatrists for their opinions. Sometimes a patient's decision to seek psychiatric help (say an alcoholic driver charged after a fatal accident who is asking for rehabilitation) may be as a result of an outstanding charge. Although many such people may be well-motivated, a proportion do seek help in order to mitigate against a harsh sentence.

The forensic history you take might be started by a question such as "Have you ever been in trouble with the police?" You will need to record all charges and convictions, together with whether this ties in with periods of mental illness. There is a high prevalence of mental illness within the UK prison system. Some 30% of prisoners have personality disorders and 4% are actively psychotic. Drug use in prison is common.

A social history needs to record where and with whom the patient is living. How do they get on with these people? A hostile environment may predispose to relapse in certain psychiatric illnesses. Are there any financial problems? Finally, unless previously recorded, how much does the patient smoke and drink? Smoking is a long-term risk factor for depression. In relapse or in times of stress or anxiety a smoker's tobacco consumption increases. Similarly alcohol consumption may rise. People with alcohol problems are notoriously evasive about exactly how much they drink. You will need to press the point. Sometimes alcoholics are reluctant themselves to face up to how much they consume. How much do they drink a day? What time of day do they start drinking? When they wake do they have a tremor that goes away with the first drink of the morning? Have they ever had the DTs (delirium tremens) or blackouts or fits? (Withdrawal fits occur in up to 10% of alcoholics.) Have they any memory problems? Failure to remember the events of the night before is sometimes referred to as a palimpsest, especially when the individual then begins to make up what they think happened the night before. These false memories are often likely things that might have happened. For example an individual may tell you a long story about doing the washing that morning and hanging it out to dry in the back garden when in fact they have been on the ward all morning. The story is 'invented' to fill the gap in their memory (which occurs because alcohol-induced brain damage has affected their ability to lay down new memories). The whole process of telling these false memories (that may appear valid to the individual) is known as confabulation. Ask also about the use of any street drugs – what types and how often and how recently? Cannabis, amphetamines, LSD and other street drugs have been associated with short- and long-term psychoses. LSD is linked to visual flashback phenomena. Amphetamines are linked to a drug-induced paranoid psychosis.

Besides street drugs you will need to take details of all currently prescribed drugs, with dosages and side-effects. Record any previous adverse reactions (e.g. acute dystonic reactions and the rare neuroleptic malignant syndrome). This can all be presented in a separate drug history.

The penultimate history item is the premorbid personality. This is an idea of the patient's personality before the first signs of any mental illness. You can ask people to describe themselves as individuals. You may need to prompt them with adjectives such as shy, or easy-going, or nervous or extrovert. You might wish to probe for hobbies or interests, favourite book or films to build up a picture of the person opposite you.

Because an individual's view of themselves is necessarily subjective, psychiatrists often ask for permission to speak to a relative or friend.

This corroborative history might shed greater light on the patient's premorbid personality and how the illness has affected them. It will allow you to check details of alcohol and drug consumption. An important point to bear in mind is that in most cases you are taking information after gaining consent from the patient. You should not offer information to the relative or friend regarding other aspects of the history or diagnosis. There is a matter of confidentiality here. (However, should the patient agree and want you to, such things may be discussed, but this probably should not arise during the history taking because your assessment and diagnosis is incomplete.)

When the history is complete there are still other components of your assessment to be done, but this is a useful time to pause and take stock of things with the patient. A useful thing to do is to summarise the history back to the patient. This has two benefits: it enables the patient to correct any mistakes you have made and therefore clarify your view of things, and it also allows the patient to feel understood by another person, sometimes for the first time in their lives. This exploration of how things have been can turn up new information and may offer some insight to the patient that they never had before. Some studies have found that patients do benefit from one-off interviews of this type. The summary is therefore an integral and vital part of the history for all concerned.

The history will allow you to generate hypotheses about what the differential diagnosis may be, but the further stages of the assessment should allow you to confirm or refute these hypotheses.

The Mental State Examination

The mental state examination seeks to:

- elicit psychological symptoms and signs
- record these symptoms and signs in a systematic way and therefore
- allow you to distinguish organic brain syndromes from other illnesses
- allow you to put evidence together to make a differential diagnosis

The mental state examination is used in every assessment, but particularly when a patient is too ill to give a history the mental state examination can be useful in making a diagnosis. The examination has a logical sequence to it, so that the first item (appearance) can give evidence which affects the conduct of the rest of the examination, for instance if the patient appears to be unconscious or is very drowsy, assessment of mood or abstract thought is rendered unreliable or even worthless.

The components of the mental state examination are:

- Appearance
- Behaviour and manner
- Speech
- Mood
- Thought
- Cognitive testing
- Insight

In the first section a brief description of the patient's appearance is made, such as 'A thin sixty-year old lady, smartly dressed, carrying a carpet bag'. The description is not intended as a judgement or to be pejorative. You should be prepared to justify everything you ever write about a patient. Having said that it is of great value to record exactly what you do see, because this will influence your diagnosis and management. If you see a 'frail elderly caucasian man, with grimy clothing and smelling of urine', then all these points may have some relevance – this appearance might suggest self-neglect, which can be a feature of general ill-health, depression, or dementia. Other more bizarre features of appearance will need documentation; e.g. ' a twenty-four year old man, wearing few clothes and with his head in a skull-cap of tin-foil, allegedly "to keep out the cosmic rays" ', or 'a large forty-year old lady, dressed only in a thin night-dress, standing in casualty, with her make-up over-liberally applied, and waving a bag of pig's trotters'. The former bizarre description accurately described a young man suffering from schizophrenia who had survived alone in a flat for two months eating raw pigeons, while the latter neatly fitted a lady with an acute episode of mania who had just been shopping in St John's market. She had not felt the need to dress that morning and had grown tired of carefully applying her make-up.

We try and separate out behaviour and manner from appearance. The patient's manner may be altogether appropriate to the interview situation: he or she may sit quietly, answering each question carefully enough. Other patients may pace the room in an agitated way whilst the doctor tries to persuade them to stay in the room to answer more questions. Patients might leap out of their chair suddenly at the behest of unseen voices, or they may be too preoccupied with visual hallucinations to concentrate on the doctor's questions. Some patients may appear unduly still, with their eyes unmoving and their limbs held tensely – these may be catatonic patients whose limbs if moved by the doctor may have increased tone and be put into unusual postures (*waxy flexibility* or *cereas flexibilitas*) which may then be held for minutes or hours (*preservation of posture*). Alternatively the patient may be mute and still because they have psychomotor retardation, as in depression – this lacks the features of increased tone and abnormal posturing. It may be appropriate to include other movement disorders under behaviour and manner – psychotropic drugs sometimes cause restlessness (*akathisia*) or acute dystonic reactions (torticollis, oculogyric crises etc.) or late-onset rhythmic involuntary lipsmacking, abnormal tongue movements, limb athetoses, and truncal movements (*tardive dyskinesias*). Patients who mimic your every move are showing *echopraxia*.

In manner patients are usually co-operative. Record this. Also try and record how well you got on with the patient in terms of rapport. Could you establish rapport with the patient? Could you both maintain eye contact, or did the patient look down at the floor throughout the interview and answer questions reluctantly or not at all? Patients may also be over-friendly in manner (disinhibited as in mania) or over-hostile (hostility may arise because patients are irritated with you or afraid of you – manic patients can be frustrated if you do not follow their fast thinking and paranoid patients may be suspicious of your motives and feel you are part of 'the plot').

The speech of the patient may be totally spontaneous or may occur only when you ask questions. The answers to questions are usually relevant, but may be wildly off the point. Sometimes all the patient's speech is spontaneous and irrelevant and any intervention by the doctor is unheeded.

Answers to questions that begin relevantly but drift from the point may be termed circumstantial speech; e.g in answer to a question about their mother's age at death: "*Well, she died young, not to say tragically, through an accident, I think there are too many accidents now. They're becoming more and more common. It's a violent world. Look at the troubles in Northern Ireland ...*". There is a conversational logic to this kind of speech, but it is difficult to focus in history-taking; the actual information that the patient's mother died at forty-five is never given. Alternatively answers to questions may be given in the minutest detail: "*my normal working day? I get up at 7.36, and wash in the bathroom whilst listening to the Today programme on Radio 4, I try not to cut myself while I shave. I shave with a razor. I like it better than an electric shaver. Then I get dressed in the clothes my wife has put out for me the night before. I like a newly ironed shirt every morning. Then I go downstairs and have two pieces of toast and a mug of freshly-brewed coffee . . .".* This kind of speech is over-inclusive – there is just too much information. Other speech types include tangential speech, which veers markedly away from the topic under discussion and may be a feature of thought disordered speech. In mania speech may be pressured – the speech is rapid and crammed with ideas that tumble over one another to be expressed. In schizophrenia and some organic disorders there may be perseverative features – the rhythmic repetition of the last words you said – known as *echolalia*, or the last syllable – *palilalia*.

Speech may be slowed down and monotonous (*psychomotor retardation in depression*). Speech disorders also include the results of brain damage (e.g. due to cerebrovascular ischaemia) which may produce dysarthrias, expressive and receptive dysphasias, and lesser word-finding difficulties.

The evidence accrued through looking at appearance, behaviour, manner and speech can be used to build up an idea about the patient's mood. Their affect during the interview may have been one of sadness or elation. The affect may have remained the same throughout the interview or it may have modulated in response to your questions (it is normal for people to be sad when recalling past traumas and happy when sharing a joke), but when affect changes suddenly and repeatedly without due cause this is known as lability of affect, which is sometimes a feature of organic brain damage. A patient's affect seems incongruous if it does not match the topic being discussed, e.g. laughter when discussing their mother's death. In patients with severe depression it may be difficult to see their affect, because they are psychomotor retarded. The severely depressed person's face may lack emotional expression, sometimes called flattened affect. In schizophrenia the patient may complain that they never feel highs or lows in their mood (blunted affect).

Using what you have found during the preceding assessment you can now build up an 'objective' view of the patient's mood, with the evidence to back this up. Ask the patient for their 'subjective' view of their mood and record this. A suitable question might be: "Can you tell me how you've been feeling, in your mood or in your spirits over the past few days or weeks?" You might like to give prompts such as "High or low? Sad or happy?" If they give a reply of sad or happy try and gauge whether this has been excessive: e.g. "How sad?" or "The saddest you've ever been?" And always probe here (in all patients) for any suicidal ideation, "Have you ever felt life was not worth living? Have you felt like this recently?" And if the answers are "yes", then ask, "Have you thought of doing anything about that? Have you got any plans to harm yourself? How would you kill yourself? When would you do it? What might stop you doing that?"

Also record again any biological features of mood disturbance: sleep abnormalities (initial insomnia, waking and early morning wakening), poor appetite, weight loss (exactly how much?), diurnal mood variation (depressed people sometimes feel worst in the morning and brighten through the day), altered sexual drive and constipation.

In the section on thought we are concerned with two main headings: form and content. The form of thought may be reflected by speech. Thus if speech is thought-disordered it may be reasonable to assume that thought (which occurs before speech) is similarly disordered. Thoughts may also be pressured, which may lead to pressure of speech, or they may be dominated by intrusive thoughts (as in obsessive compulsive disorder), or may exhibit flights of ideas (as in mania), or sudden unpleasant gaps (as in thought blocking in schizophrenia). In the content of thought you might ask for the main thoughts that dominate a person's recent thinking life: "What kind of things do you think about most?"; "What kind of things do you worry about nowadays?" Record any worries, preoccupations, intrusive thoughts, over-valued ideas or delusions. Under thought content you may also record any abnormal experiences such as hallucinatory experiences or thought interference (withdrawal, insertion, or broadcasting).

In cognition we are interested in eliciting signs that may point to an organic psychiatric disease. If consciousness is diminished or 'clouded' then this may mean that hallucinations are the product of a delirious state (acute organic brain syndrome) as in pyrexia or temporal lobe epilepsy. If there are memory problems on cognitive testing then it may be that there is a dementing process at work.

A basic scheme for cognitive testing might be:

- *Orientation* – normally in daytime people are aware of the time, the place they are in and the people they are with. In organic brain syndrome this orientation to time, place and person is gradually lost. It is possible to be disorientated just in time or disorientated in all three. Ask for the current date (day, date, month, year) and the time of day. Ask for the place ("Where are we now?"); find out if the patient knows which ward, hospital, or clinic they are in. Finally do they know who you are, or do they imagine you to be a priest or a social worker (given that you have introduced yourself properly at some time during the interview)?

- *Attention and Concentration* – An inability to focus attention may be seen in agitated depression, anxiety, mania or organic syndromes. Tests which can be used include: "Please say the months of the year for me in reverse order, that is working backwards from December through to January . . ." or "Please say the days of the week in reverse order, staring with Sunday and working back to Monday", or "Please take seven away from 100, now carry on taking 7 away from that, and again . . ." (known as 'serial sevens') or "Please take 3 away from 21 and keep on taking 3 away until there is nothing left" ('serial threes'). Other tests may include digit spans – seeing how many numbers an individual can repeat back to you in sequence or reverse sequence, e.g. 364 . . . 463, 7924 . . . 4297. These tests help you assess attention, but do involve other skills too, so that if these other skills are lost then it may appear that attention is poor when it is not. For example, if someone is poor at maths or has a specific brain defect which causes dyscalculia (a parietal lobe deficit) then serial sevens or serial threes will not produce useful results.

- *Memory* – Some people define short-term memory as everything remembered up to three minutes ago, and everything retained beyond three minutes or so as medium or long-term memory. Definitions of short and long-term memory are contentious though and you will observe that different psychiatrists and psychologists have different ideas about this. In a basic cognitive screen we are interested in fairly crude tests of memory function – short-term testing may involve asking someone to remember a new name and address. "I would like you to listen to and remember a new name and address I am going to say to you. I will repeat it until you are happy that you have got it in mind." The name and address may have seven components, say. See initially how many times you have to repeat the name and address before the individual can repeat it back word-perfect (i.e. how many times does it take before they register the address). then ask them to recall the address at fixed intervals (thirty seconds, one minute, three minutes and five minutes, say), and then record how many components they can give back to you:

	Thirty seconds	One minute	Three minutes	Five minutes
Number of Address Components	7/7	6/7	4/7	2/7

This gives you an 'objective' measure of memory function which you can use for later comparison. Other short-term tests might include giving a list of five different objects and asking the individual to repeat these back to you at certain times. You will also need to get an idea of long-term memory function – can the individual recall important personal dates (e.g. birthday and anniversaries) – only useful if you have an objective source to check these with – or the dates of important historical events (date of Second World War, death of Churchill, date of first moon landing etc.). You can sometimes ask for the names of five flowers, five animals or five capital cities. Short-term memory function deteriorates first in dementia syndromes, but all these memory tests may be affected in severe dementia or by mental retardation.

- *Specific tests of cerebral lobe function* – if the cognitive screening has been normal up to now, then it is probably not of use to probe further into cerebral lobe function However, if a dementia syndrome seems likely then some simple tests may be useful in determining whether there is frontal or parietal lobe damage.

A simple test for frontal lobe damage seeks to assess whether there are any perseverative tendencies. The patient is asked to copy a rhythmically changing line pattern:

In some frontal lobe deficits the patient may perseverate as follows:

Paper tests for parietal lobe damage may seek to assess whether there is a constructional apraxia. When asked to copy a line drawing of a house, the copy may be 'exploded', or there may be sensory inattention to one side of the diagram:

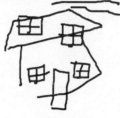
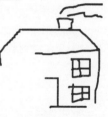

Normal copy   'exploded'   'sensory inattention'

- *Abstract thought* – in schizophrenia and in some mental retardation the capacity for abstract thinking may be reduced, so that concrete thinking is prevalent. When asked to interpret a proverb or saying such as 'a rolling stone gathers no moss' the concrete interpretation would be 'because the moss can't stick'. Test for abstract thought may therefore include asking for the meaning of proverbs or for asking for similarities between things such as a banana and an apple (correct answer – 'both fruits' or 'both living things') or a car and a lorry, or for differences between things like a lake and a river or a child and a dwarf. Such tests may also provoke thought disorder in some predisposed individuals.

Finally, the mental state examination seeks to assess 'insight' – whether an individual sees their problems as being due to ill-health, and if so being treatable by doctors, and if so whether treatable by drugs. Psychotic illnesses often rob patients of insight so that they feel their voices are normal, or naturally derived, or attributable to some alien authority rather than a treatable illness. If they make this assumption about their psychotic experiences and delusions then it is logical to think that doctors cannot help, and that drug treatment therefore offers no logical benefit to them. In this way lack of insight may affect patient compliance with treatment, which is refused, condemning the psychiatrically unwell to permanent ill-health. Insight is therefore about how the patient sees their predicament and is a complex construct.

Physical Examination and Investigations

Psychiatrists are first and foremost doctors, trained in diagnosis, and keen to exclude any treatable physical illness which may present with psychological symptoms. A routine physical examination of cardio-vascular, respiratory, abdominal and nervous systems is therefore essential in all patients. Organic causes of psychiatric illness which may picked up in this way might include: focal CNS lesions, subdural haematomas, systemic lupus erythematosus, hyperthyroidism, hypothyroidism, diabetes mellitus, Addison's disease, Cushing's disease, hypertension, renal and liver failure, phaeochromocytomas, tuberous sclerosis, syphilis, bronchial and gastric carcinomas, stigmata of alcoholic liver disease, features of mental retardation syndromes (e.g. Down's, fragile-X) and numerous others.

Investigations similarly may usefully include FBC (various

anaemias may present with dementia-like pictures, raised MCV in alcoholism), LFTs (raised in alcoholism), TFTs, serum B_{12} and folate, urea and electrolytes, syphilis screening tests, drug screening tests (street drugs may induce psychotic reactions), chest and skull X-rays, EEG (to detect focal lesions and epileptic phenomena), CT/NMR scans, and more specialist tests e.g. cortisol levels, dexamethasone suppression tests, homovanillic acid urine tests and serum copper tests (for Wilson's disease).

Other investigations may include social, occupational and psychological investigations. Social investigations (if consented to) may include discussions with family and friends, requests to schools for information on progress and abilities, home visits and the like. Occupational therapists may assist not only with rehabilitation, but also functional assessments (how well people can manage their home life and plan their daily activities). Psychologists can sometimes help with specific neuropsychological tests of brain function, and personality and IQ testing.

Putting the Information Together

At the end of the assessment the doctor pulls together the major findings from the history, mental state, physical examination and investigations into a summary. Sometimes the summary is built into a 'formulation' which also includes a differential diagnosis and a tentative management plan and prognosis. The differential diagnosis should include the most likely diagnoses, headed by the most likely of all, together with evidence, extracted from the assessment interview, to support or refute each diagnosis. Using the differential diagnosis, the doctor can then, and only then, reasonably construct a management plan and prognosis which can be appended to the formulation.

In making your differential diagnosis you may wish to consider four 'levels' of illness in a sort of diagnostic sieve. The first level to consider is organic: specifically, ask yourself if there is any organic illness that might present with such features. This must be included in your differential diagnosis and steps must be taken to exclude treatable organic illness. It makes little sense to embark on psychological methods of treatment without treating underlying organic causes. The second level is psychotic illness, by which we mean illnesses with psychotic features (such as hallucinations and delusions) which are not caused by gross organic disorder (such as delirium or intracerebral tumours or infarctions). Such psychotic illnesses are schizophrenia and severe affective disorders like major depressive disorders and mania.

The third level is neurotic illness which encompasses minor disturbances of mood, anxiety disorders, phobias and eating disorders. Such illnesses may be very disabling, but they lack psychotic features. Finally, the fourth area to consider involves the personality. People's personalities differ to a greater or lesser extent. When those differences are marked, persistent and damaging to the individual or society, they are termed personality disorders. Some personality disorders may mimic other psychiatric illness, but it is worth bearing in mind that, just as all personality types can become physically ill, then all personality types can suffer from psychiatric illness. It would be unethical to deny treatment to someone purely on the basis that they had a personality disorder.

Classification

Separate chapters in this series will discuss specific disorders in more detail, but for now a summary of classification may be useful.

Classifying diseases helps doctors to recognise clinically similar illnesses in people and enables research, particularly in terms of what causes those illnesses and what cures them. In psychiatry, large groups have met to define illness categories, and currently there are two broad classification systems in use. The European and world-wide system is the International Classification of Diseases, 10th version (ICD-10), and the American system is the Diagnostic and Statistical Manual, 3rd version – revised (DSM-III-R). There is substantial overlap between them. When you make a diagnosis according to the criteria for each disease in these classifications then other clinicians will know what you mean when you diagnose schizophrenia. A few decades ago there was considerable disagreement between American and UK psychiatrists as to how schizophrenia could be diagnosed. Different criteria were used in the different countries, leading to an apparent over-diagnosis of schizophrenia in America, compared to the UK. Now relatively similar standard criteria are used in both countries and the mismatch in rates of diagnosis has evened out.

A useful thumbnail classification to have in mind when interviewing a patient is the one in the psychiatric 'sieve' above: organic, psychotic, neurotic and personality. However, in making a diagnosis the following classification may be of use. Although one diagnosis may take precedence, remember that several conditions may be present.

ICD-10
(Adopted as a standard by the World Health Organisation in 1992)

F00–F09
Organic mental disorders
Examples:
Dementia in Alzheimer's disease – early or late onset
Vascular dementia (acute, multi-infarct, subcortical types)
Dementia in Pick's disease, Creutzfeldt–Jakob disease, Huntington's chorea, Parkinson's disease, and HIV disease
Delirium (an acute organic brain syndrome with disorientation and clouding of consciousness)
Organic hallucinosis (e.g. caused by TLE), organic mood disorders (e.g. in Cushing's syndrome), organic anxiety disorders (e.g. in phaeochromocytoma)
Organic personality disorder (e.g. frontal lobe tumours which may disorganise personality), post-encephalitic syndromes and post-concussional syndromes.]

F10–F19
Mental and behavioural disorders due to psychoactive substance abuse
Covers alcohol, opioids, cannabinoids, sedatives, hypnotics, cocaine, caffeine, amphetamines, other hallucinogens, tobacco, solvents, other drugs
May include harmful use, dependence, withdrawal states, psychotic disorders (e.g. delirium tremens and LSD experiences), amnesic syndromes (e.g. Wernicke-Korsakoff syndrome) and residual effects (e.g. LSD flashbacks).

F20–F29
Schizophrenia, schizotypal and delusional disorders
Schizophrenia (paranoid, hebephrenic, catatonic, undifferentiated, residual)
Schizotypal disorder (lacks the full psychotic features of schizophrenia – often seen as more of an extreme of personality with unusual eccentric ideation – magical thinking)
Persistent delusional disorders (e.g. monodelusional psychoses where the individual wrongly believes they are, say, infested by some insect, but have no other psychotic features.
Schizoaffective disorder – rare category with strong features of both affective illness and schizophrenia.

F30–F39
Mood (affective) disorders
Manic episode (hypomania is a lesser form of mania and probably more common, mania without psychotic features, mania with psychotic features)
Bipolar affective disorder (evidence of both hypomanic/manic and depressive episodes at some stage in a person's life)
Depressive episodes (mild, moderate and severe without depressive symptoms and severe with psychotic symptoms)
Recurrent mood disorders
Persistent mood disorders (cyclothymia, dysthymia)

F40–F48
Neurotic, stress-related and somatoform disorders
Phobic anxiety disorders (agoraphobia, social phobias, specific phobias)
Anxiety disorders (panic disorder, generalised anxiety disorder)
Obsessive–compulsive disorder (obsessional thoughts or ruminations, compulsive acts and obsessional rituals)
Reactions to severe stress and adjustment disorders
Dissociative (conversion) disorders – where some internal conflict or anxiety is converted into

other symptoms such as classical Freudian hysterical paralysis (dissociative amnesias, dissociative fugues, trance and possession states, dissociative convulsions, dissociative anaesthesia)
Somatoform disorders – somatising anxiety into any physical symptom
Depersonalisation–derealisation syndrome

F50–F59
Behavioural syndromes associated with physiological disturbances and physical factors

Eating disorders (anorexia nervosa, bulimia nervosa and others)
Nonorganic sleep disorders (where organic causes have been excluded – insomnia, hypersomnia, somnambulism, night terrors, nightmares)
Sexual dysfunction (not caused by organic disorder or disease); includes loss of sexual desire, sexual aversion, failure of genital response, orgasmic dysfunction, premature ejaculation, nonorganic vaginismus, nonorganic dyspareunia, excessive sexual drive and others
Mental and behavioural disorders of the puerperium
Abuse of non-dependence-producing substances (like laxatives, analgesics, antacids, vitamins etc.)

F60–F69
Disorders of adult personality and behaviour

Personality disorders (including paranoid, schizoid, dissocial, borderline, histrionic, anankastic, avoidant, dependent, and other types)
Enduring personality change after catastrophic experience or psychiatric illness
Pathological gambling, firesetting, stealing, hair-pulling.
Transsexualism, dual-role transvestism
Sexual preference disorders – fetishism, exhibitionism, voyeurism, paedophilia, sado-masochism etc.
Factitious disorder (intentional feigning of symptoms or disabilities), sometimes also called Munchausen's syndrome

F70–F79
Mental retardation

Mild, moderate, severe and profound

F80–F89
Disorders of psychological development

Developmental disorders of speech, receptive and expressive language disorders, specific arithmetical disorders
Childhood autism, Rett's syndrome, Asperger's syndrome

F90–F98
Behavioural and emotional disorders with onset usually occurring in childhood and adolescence

Hyperkinetic disorders, conduct disorders, emotional disorders, tic disorders, non-organic enuresis, non-organic encopresis, pica, stereotyped movement disorders, stuttering

F99
Unspecified mental disorder

Self-Assessment Tests

1. **In the following mental state abnormalities:**

A thought blocking is where alien thoughts are inserted into the patient's mind to block their own thoughts
B perseveration is a typical consequence of temporal lobe lesions
C flight of ideas implies an acceleration of the flow of thinking
D intrusive thoughts are incorrect, unreasonable, bizarre ideas held with absolute conviction
E thought echo is a neurotic symptom

2. **Frontal lobe syndrome is associated with:**

A absence of the grasp reflex
B lack of initiative
C dressing dyspraxia
D hemisomatoagnosia
E impaired judgement

3. **Depersonalisation:**

A can occur in schizophrenia
B is when the world around feels unreal but the self feels the same as usual
C is sometimes a symptom of temporal lobe epilepsy
D is usually indicative of psychotic illness
E is a very rare human experience

4. **The following disorders are classified as ICD-10 mood disorders:**

A schizotypal disorder
B hemisomatoagnosia
C dysthymia
D cyclothymia
E Rett's syndrome

5. **Recognized features of temporal lobe dysfunction include:**

A constructional dyspraxia
B pressure of speech
C memory disturbance
D Broca's expressive dysphasia
E hallucinations

6. Characteristic features of anorexia nervosa include:

A morbid fear of weight gain
B altered body image
C binge-eating
D loss of secondary sexual characteristics
E dysmenorrhoea

7. Types of delusion occurring in schizophrenia include:

A paranoid
B auditory
C religious
D olfactory
E grandiose

8. Please read this case history and answer the questions that follow:

John Murdstone came into the surgery to ask for bowel surgery. He said that his bowels had become blocked over the last two months. He was convinced that he had cancer of the colon which had eliminated his lower bowel and that he had only a few weeks to live. His general practitioner could find no symptoms or signs to confirm any evidence of bowel obstruction and Mr Murdstone appeared to be a fit man in his early forties. There was no history of gastrointestinal problems, but Mr Murdstone had an episode of depression four years ago, after losing his job. His doctor tried to reassure him, but Mr Murdstone was adamant. His bowels had 'shrivelled away with cancer' so that his lower bowel had 'disappeared'. It was a 'judgement' on him, which he thoroughly deserved. Mr Murdstone felt that he was responsible for the level of unemployment in the country, because he was not being efficient at work. He could see no future for himself or his young family, and felt that he and they would be better off when he was dead.

(a) What mental state abnormalities could be present?
(b) What aspects of his history contribute to the differential diagnosis?
(c) What 'danger signals' are present in the mental state?

Self-assessment: Answers

1. A=F, B=F, C=T, D=F, E=F.
2. A=F. B=T, C=F, D=F, E=T.
3. A=T, B=F, C=T, D=F, E=F.
4. A=F, B=F, C=T, D=T, E=F.
5. A=F, B=F, C=T, D=F, E=T.
6. A=T, B=T, C=F, D=F, E=F.
7. A=T, B=F, C=T, D=F, E=T.
8. (a) nihilistic delusions and delusions of guilt
   (b) a past history of depressive illness
   (c) the belief that he and his family would be better off if he were dead – he is a clear suicidal risk.

Further reading

Fish, F. (Edited by Max Hamilton) (1977) Clinical Psychopathology. Bristol, Wright.

Jaspers, K. (1959) General Psychopathology. Manchester University Press.

Sims, A. (1988) Symptoms in the Mind. London, Bailliere Tindall.

World Health Organisation. (1992) The ICD-10 Classification of Mental and Behavioural Disorders. Geneva, WHO.

Danger Signals and the Mental Health Act

In considering danger we must look at dangers that patients create for other people and the dangers they create for themselves. Much danger arises from extreme affect such as severe depression or fear, or abnormal thoughts such as a delusional system. An example of danger arising from fear is the sudden attack from a patient in an acute confusional state who misconstrues the world around him. A disorientated hypoxic patient might mistake the GP on a night visit, listening to his chest with a stethoscope, for a mugger about to garrotte him. Depression may lead to suicide as a result of hopelessness or delusional thought, e.g. a seventy-year old man who wrongly thinks he is guilty of a serious crime. Depression may occasionally lead to homicidal behaviour for 'altruistic' rather than aggressive or selfish reasons, e.g. the depressed post-natal mother who feels that the world is such a dreadful place that she would kill her young family rather than let them grow up and 'suffer so' in later life. Patients with schizophrenia may hear voices telling them to harm themselves or others and may ultimately succumb to the hallucinatory commands. Paranoid schizophrenia may involve systematised persecutory delusions which require the sufferer to kill a third party. Such third parties are most commonly close relatives (usually the mother), but may involve 'distant' third parties such as the Prime Minister, or the Pope.

So, what signals should alert the GP to possible danger to the patient or others? Such danger signals include:

- depressed affect (always probe for suicidal ideation)
- disorientation and fearful misinterpretation of events
- extreme anxiety and concern for the safety of self or others
- persecutory delusions
- disinhibition and irritable hypomania
- hallucinatory commands
- a past history of 'dangerousness'
- a history of assaultativeness

- previous firesetting behaviour
- disinhibition due to alcohol or drugs

Certain precautions should be taken with potentially violent patients. It is difficult to give a complete list or to tailor such a list to circumstances. Some of the seemingly most dramatic seeming situations can resolve very quickly and satisfactorily and some of the apparently most benign situations can escalate nastily out of control. Check through the following list and see which precautions you are prepared to take routinely:

- *never* interview potentially violent patients alone in a place where there is no way you can call for immediate help
- reduce their level of fear (making an attack on you less likely) by interviewing with the door slightly ajar (so they don't feel trapped – and neither do you), by getting on the same eye level as them, by looking and sounding 'non-threatening'
- acknowledge their anger/fear – get them to explain it to you so that you can defuse it and correct misunderstandings
- ensure that physical support (physical restraint or sedation) is rapidly available to you if you should call out – arrange a pre-determined signal to call for help – and make sure there are adequate numbers of staff to help you. Call for police back-up if unsure
- if disorientation is at the root of their fear ensure the interview room is well-lit
- ensure that no weapons are available to the individual, and ensure that your own clothing/instruments cannot be used against you – e.g. remove any ties or scarves before commencing the interview
- ensure that you do not allow less trained staff to take on more risks on your behalf than you know are safe

Suicide

One of the explicit aims of *The Health of the Nation* is to reduce the suicide rate. Generally the incidence of suicide rises with age, but is higher in males than females at all ages, unlike the incidence of deliberate self harm. Half of all male suicides now occur in the over 50s. Suicide is less common in those who are married than in the unmarried, and highest of all in the divorced, separated and widowed.

Socioeconomic class also has an influence, with rates highest in class V and lowest in classes II and III. Some occupations with high risk rates include lawyers, writers, nurses, farmers, hotel and bar workers and doctors.

Other risk factors for suicide include a family history of suicide and immigrant status. Rates are highest in urban rather than rural areas and peak in autumn.

Unemployment is linked to suicide but a causal link is not so clear – it may be, for instance, that mental disorder increases the risk of unemployment as well as suicide. Whereas females more commonly resort to self poisoning, males tend to use more violent methods, such as hanging, shooting and drowning. Poisoning with car exhaust fumes is becoming increasingly common in young males.

Suicide in mental disorders

Of those who have had a major depressive disorder, 15% will go on eventually to kill themselves and are more likely to be:

- older
- male
- single
- living alone

and to have:

- hopelessness
- anhedonia (loss of pleasure in things)
- loss of interest
- insomnia
- self-neglect
- more severe depression
- a previous suicide attempt
- mood cycling

The Mental Health Act (1983) and the General Practitioner

The 1983 Mental Health Act may involve general practitioners in providing assessments on their patients in the community and in hospital. The GP has a unique role in these assessments in that they may have first-hand knowledge of their patient derived from many years' knowledge of the patient and their family. The GP will be able to make a comparison with the patient's everyday mental state and level of functioning. Section 12 approved GPs may be called upon to provide assessments on patients other than their own. Assessment fees are payable, usually via social services, whether the GP is approved or not. Fees should be paid whether or not the GP goes on to complete a section recommendation. If you are asked to provide an assessment keep a confidential record of the patient's name, address, the date of the assessment, who requested the assessment, where it took place, your travelling expenses, and the attending social worker's name. The claim for the section should be made on your behalf by the attending social worker (check that this is so at the time of the assessment) even if the social worker does fill in the paperwork on your behalf, you may need to check and follow up the claim and will need the above information to do so.

What Mental Health Act sections involve general practitioners?

The sections that commonly involve GPs are sections 2 and 3. GPs may be asked to provide a second medical recommendation on their own patients in casualty or in hospital. Section 2 is intended as an assessment section and lasts for 28 days. There is a provision for assessment *and* treatment during this time. Section 3 is intended as a treatment section for patients who have an established diagnosis and where there is some formulated management plan. It lasts for six months, in recognition of the fact that treatment for mental illness may need to be prolonged. Patients can be, and usually are, discharged at any time before the expiry of these sections. Patients have the right of appeal against both sections.

Both sections require two medical recommendations – one from a doctor approved under section 12 of the Act as having special experience in the diagnosis of mental illness, and one from a doctor with prior knowledge of the patient. Once the recommendations are completed an approved social worker can make an application to the managers of the hospital for the compulsory admission/assessment/treatment under the particular section. The application can be made by the nearest relative, but in practice this usually involves the social worker.

The GP usually has to ensure by interview that the patient has a mental disorder, that the patient's health, or the safety of the patient or others is in some way compromised, and that the patient is not consenting to voluntary admission. It is usual to take into account any relevant history, for instance, a recent attack on a third party, or a recent suicide attempt. The interview may be jointly conducted. The medical recommendations may be completed separately or as a 'joint recommendation'. In either case there should be consultation between the doctors and between the doctors and the approved social worker.

GPs may find themselves trying to initiate section proceedings themselves in the community. It helps if a bed has been identified by the GP at a neighbouring hospital. The GP should then usually contact the district social service team or the emergency social service team (if after office hours or at the weekend). The social service team should then be able to arrange a second medical opinion by an approved doctor. Once the section is completed the social worker has a duty to convey the patient to hospital.

What happens if things don't go according to plan?

One of the problems with drafting legislation such as the Mental Health Act is that the Act needs to fit a variety of situations. Those who have been in the position of trying to initiate section proceedings will appreciate that there are more variables in the system than anybody could legislate for. Patients will disappear out of the back door as one arrives, or barricade themselves inside their houses and refuse interviews. Social workers and psychiatrists may be as difficult to contact as the dead. Hospital beds may be as rare as rain in the desert. In such circumstances you can only do your best (and keep a purely factual account of events – just in case).

Sections of the Act that try to take some account of the unpredictability of real life include sections 4, 135 and 136.

Section 4 covers an emergency admission for assessment. It can provide for admission with the recommendation of one doctor and the application of a social worker. The section lasts for 72 hours. It can be useful where situations are acute and no second doctor can be obtained in time. Section 136 allows a police officer to remove someone they suspect of having a mental disorder from a public place to a 'place of safety' which may be a police station or an accident and emergency department. The section may last 72 hours, or until the individual is seen by an approved doctor and an approved social worker. Section 135 allows police officers to take someone that they and a magistrate suspect of having a mental disorder from private property and remove them to a 'place of safety'.

Where can I find out more about the Act?

It is impossible to cover all aspects of mental health law here, so we would recommend that you research further. The Mental Health Act (1983) itself is obtainable from branches of the HMSO, as is the current *Code of Practice*, published by the Department of Health and the Welsh Office (1993). Separate legislation governs the Republic of Ireland and Scotland.

If you believe that you may have enough experience in psychiatry to allow you to become Section 12 approved, seek the advice of the Regional Health Authority who may be able to advise you on the local procedures for obtaining or renewing approval.

What about the future?

Following recent difficulties with the Government *Care in the Community* scheme, there is increased emphasis on aftercare. That the Act seeks to treat those who are ill and lack insight as well as those who are ill and a danger to themselves and others is being highlighted. Similarly hospitals and social services are being asked to pay more attention to the provision of co-ordinated aftercare for previously sectioned patients. GPs may be asked to participate in so-called section 117 meetings where these care plans are theoretically thrashed out and key workers appointed. At the time of writing it seems possible that the Act will be amended. The possibility of community treatment orders has been raised.

Other Mental Health Legislation

Changes to the Mental Health Act are necessary (Eastman, 1994), particularly to effect adequate psychiatric care in the community and simultaneously to protect civil liberties. Principles contained within the 1983 Act lag behind later legislation such as the NHS and Community Care Act, 1990. Putting ethical considerations on one side for a moment, there is no real provision for compulsory medication within the community in the 1983 Act. Mental Health care for children is a problem area. Rarely, compulsory treatment is given to a child under a section of the Mental Health Act, but there is a need for specific consideration, although the Children Act, 1989 has some overlap in this area. Radical reform of the Mental Health Act (1983) is therefore being considered.

The NHS and Community Care Act, 1990 sought to enact some ideas contained within the white papers, *Working for Patients* and *Caring for*

People. The main thrust of the sections dealing with community care was to give the main co-ordinating role as 'lead agency' to local social service authorities, who are charged with providing needs assessments for patients. However, having identified needs, whether they are met is another matter, and whether there is any legal obligation to fulfil those needs is unclear as yet.

What goes into an assessment?

A social worker fills in a form with various headings, accompanied by a checklist in certain areas. A specialist evaluation can be requested to accompany the form. During the process the patient and carers should be consulted (and the carer may have an assessment in their own right). Advocacy services can represent patients if they feel that they would like additional support.

A model for an assessment of need is the Camberwell Assessment of Need (CAN), developed at the Institute of Psychiatry, that covers the following areas:

Accommodation	Safety to Others
Occupation	Money
Psychotic Symptoms	Childcare
Psychological Distress	Physical health
Information about condition	Alcohol
and treatment	Basic Education
Non-prescribed drugs	Company
Food and Meals	Telephone
Household Skills	Public Transport
Self-care and Presentation	Benefits
Safety to Self	Sexual Relations

The well-meaning principles behind mental health policy sometimes have difficulty being translated into economic reality. A ring-fenced transfer of funds from the area of health budgets to social services budgets is problematic. The sums likely to be involved are considerable. The 1980s saw a decrease in hospital bed provision for the long-term elderly. This, together with demographic changes, saw expenditure on residential and nursing home care rise from £10 million in 1979 to £1 billion in 1989 (Secretaries of State, 1989).

A number of initiatives are required to make the reforms work – district health authorities and GP fundholders need to partner each other in commissioning community services. This will ensure that gaps in service provision are filled. The next two sections of this book look at how mental health problems can be identified from assessments and describe what services may be available. The reforms offer an opportunity to meet identified needs with newly developed and more user-friendly services, but insufficient overall funding will potentially destroy the strategy altogether.

References

Eastman, N. (1994) Mental health law: civil liberties and the principle of reciprocity. British Medical Journal, 308, 43–45.

Secretaries of State for Health, Social Security, Wales, and Scotland. (1989) Caring for People, Community Care in the Next Decade and Beyond. London, HMSO

Secretaries of State for Health, Wales, Northern Ireland and Scotland. (1989) Working for Patients. London, HMSO.

Self-Assessment Tests

1. **Section Two (MHA, 1983):**
A   lasts for six months
B   allows for assessment but not compulsory treatment in hospital
C   has no provision for appeal by the patient
D   can be applied for by the nearest relative
E   can be renewed *ad infinitum*

2. **In the 1983 Mental Health Act:**
A   Section 136 allows a police constable to remove a mentally disordered person from that person's home
B   Section 4 lasts for six days
C   Section 3 requires the recommendations of two doctors and two social workers
D   Section 4 requires the recommendation of just one doctor who *must* be approved
E   there is a section which allows psychosurgery to be performed without the patient's consent

Answers

1. A=F, B=F, C=F, D=T, E=F
2. A=F, B=F, C=F, D=F, E=F

Mental Health Screening

The identified cases of mental disorder treated by psychiatric services represent only the tip of the iceberg of mental distress. Most of the community's mental illness remains undiagnosed and untreated, although it most certainly is suffered by those affected and their families. In a longitudinal study of mental health in the community in Liverpool only 4% of elderly people with depressive illness were treated (Copeland et al., 1992).

Before patients can be treated they must be diagnosed. Before they can be diagnosed they must be in touch with some medical agency. Before people contact a doctor they must recognise that they have an illness that can be treated. Although people may suffer with mental illness they are also notoriously bad at recognising their symptoms as an illness at all. Symptoms may be wrongly wholly attributed to a physical illness, or to some recent untoward life event (although physical health and life events are major aetiological factors in mental disorder). Screening for mental disorders would seek to pick up unidentified cases of mental disorder that can be treated, but exactly which illnesses should be screened for, how and by whom, and with what end result in mind is a matter for some debate. Should doctors screen using screening instruments, or should they leave such screening devices to other health personnel? Should highly trained doctors need to use screening instruments at all?

Goldberg and Huxley (1992) identified five levels of care and four filters between these levels:

		Psychological symptoms
Level One	The Community	260–315/1000 per year
Filter One (Illness behaviour)		
Level Two	Attenders in Primary Care	230/1000 per year
Filter Two (Ability of GP to detect disorder)		
Level Three	Cases detected by doctors	101.5/1000 per year
Filter Three (Referral to mental illness services)		
Level Four	Attenders in psychiatric services	23.5/1000 per year
Filter Four (Admission to psychiatric beds)		
Level Five	Psychiatric in-patients	5.71/1000 per year

Goldberg and Huxley's filter and level model clearly illustrates the point that the majority of morbidity is undiagnosed and untreated – but what form does this morbidity take?

Epidemiological studies suggest that the bulk of this morbidity is probably 'minor' psychological distress taking the form of anxiety disorders or adjustment reactions (which may affect as much as 20–30% of the population at any one time). Even so, such minor disorders are so prevalent that they form a major cause of disability as far as society is concerned. The direct and indirect costs of such illness may be as high as £1 billion a year in the UK alone. Community studies have used instruments such as the General Health Questionnaire (GHQ) to screen for morbidity, but such instruments usually do not give precise diagnoses. Having acknowledged the prevalence of such psychological distress and its costs to the individual and society, we should ask ourselves the following:

Audit Points

- *how can minor psychological morbidity be better detected?*
- *how can this morbidity be best treated?*
- *what results or outcome measures can we use to assess the efficacy of detection and treatment?*

There are problems inherent in this approach – and these are political as much as anything, in that using medical services to address this minor psychological morbidity will divert resources away from more 'severe' mental disorders with a lower incidence, such as schizophrenia. Community Psychiatric Nurses working in some general practices spend more time with neurotic patients than with chronic psychotic patients (Wooff et al., 1986). Moving resources away from 'traditional' psychiatric patients may jeopardise the future of care in the community for rehabilitated people with chronic psychoses.

Since one of the largest barriers to primary care diagnosis occurs between Level One and Level Two, some effort must be put into raising community awareness and stimulating the sufferers to come forward and present. An alternative would be to pro-actively find cases. Such an approach has a precedent in recent initiatives to promote screening of the elderly in general practice. In terms of doctors themselves as case-finding instruments, good detectors of psychiatric morbidity tend to be empathic, are interested in psychiatry, ask questions about the patient's family and home, are self-confident, clarify complaints, have accurate psychiatric knowledge and have high academic ability (Marks et al., 1979; Goldberg et al., 1980). With these factors in mind, the first two sections on rapport and psychopathology, respectively, sought to address issues of empathic interview style and revise concepts in psychiatric diagnosis.

However, is it desirable to detect minor morbidity and attach diagnostic labels to sufferers – in other words to turn people into 'cases'? There are alternative models of re-framing people's distress and alternative sources of treatment within the community. A vast array of formal and informal counselling occurs in the community without recourse to medical diagnosis or treatment. Previous forays by doctors into the treatment of anxiety disorders (such as the once widespread prescription of benzodiazepines) are now viewed as controversial.

Perhaps one of the things that should worry us as doctors is the slight possibility that such minor illness is misdiagnosed by whatever lay person seeks to provide treatment. It is possible to conjure up images of past patients who have been treated with lengthy group analysis for anxiety which turned out to be a product of thyrotoxicosis, or given counselling for panic disorder when in fact they have been suffering with intermittent diabetic hypoglycaemia, or of other patients being given cognitive therapy when suffering from severe depressive illness.

Such misdiagnosis is less likely if patients present first to their doctor. General practices increasingly offer anxiety management groups and the services of counsellors. Even so, the unplanned expansion of general practice counsellors is a source of concern to some authorities who question the costs involved, and others who question the training of such individuals. Presumably as a result of such concern audit studies will be performed on the cost–efficacy of such interventions, and estimate the cost savings involved (for instance, do recipients of counselling services attend less often for physical investigations and treatments?). Concern will also lead to organisations seeking to standardise counsellors in terms of training and the treatments employed. Psychotherapy and counselling are considered further in Part Two.

Although providing supportive psychotherapy can be a rewarding experience for the doctor, as outlined by Balint (1964), it is unlikely that the GP will be able to afford time to formally counsel all his or her patients that might benefit by such an approach. Nevertheless, timed psychological and family interventions by the GP can be profoundly powerful and effective in the long term. GPs should have clear criteria in mind when referring patients for psychological treatment. In 'prescribing' psychotherapy GPs are, in effect, prescribing a 'drug' with its own indications, contra-indications, side-effects and addictivity. GPs therefore need to be aware of the general structure and content of such therapies, if not the specific detail discussed between therapist and patient.

The less common psychiatric illnesses such as moderate and severe depression, anorexia nervosa, bipolar affective disorder, dementia and schizophrenia may be less difficult to detect, and sufferers and their relatives may be more likely to bring the problem to the attention of their doctor. However, if the patient's insight has been lost, then even severe cases of illness may still go unpresented.

Patients with alcohol, drug and eating disorders often do not present totally out of their own choice – often more through a consequence of their behaviour. A high index of suspicion is often the best instrument in screening for these problems. It helps to attach a set of rehearsed questions to such suspicions. Kessel and Walton (1989), quoting Wilkins' 1974 work, estimate that only one-tenth of alcoholics are diagnosed as such, despite their being recognised as ill individuals. The CAGE questions (Mayfield et al., 1974) are an example of a validated screening instrument for alcoholism:

- C   have you ever felt you should CUT down on your drinking?
- A   have people ANNOYED you by criticising your drinking?
- G   have you ever felt bad or GUILTY about your drinking?
- E   have you ever had a drink first thing in the morning to steady your nerves or get rid of a hang-over (EYE-OPENER)?

Two positive answers on the CAGE are strongly suggestive of alcoholism.

The shortened Michigan Alcoholism Screening Test (MAST) is a series of 10 alternative questions (Pokorny et al., 1972).

- do you feel you are a normal drinker?
- do friends or relatives think you are a normal drinker?
- have you ever attended a meeting of Alcoholics Anonymous (AA)?
- have you ever lost friends or girl/boy friends because of drinking?
- have you ever gotten into trouble at work because of drinking?
- have you ever neglected your obligations, your family, your work for more than two days in a row because you were drinking?

- have you ever had delirium tremens (DTs), severe shaking, heard voices or seen things that weren't there after heavy drinking?
- have you ever been in a hospital because of your drinking?
- have you ever been arrested for drunk driving or driving after drinking?

To score the brief MAST, you score 2 for a negative answer to the first and second questions, and for positive answers to the remainder you score either five or two (for question 3 yes = 5, for question 4 yes = 2, and for 5,6,7,8,9 and 10 score 2,2,2,5,5,and 2 respectively for positive answers). A score above 18 indicates severe problems. Most non-alcoholics score less than 5.

Mean Cell Volume and γ-GT are possible physical tests to confirm diagnostic hypotheses.

In terms of the spectrum of eating disorders, anorexia nervosa (at one end of the spectrum), probably affects some 1–2% of adolescent women in the UK. Abnormal eating attitudes, including binge eating and vomiting, may be present in up to 4–5% of young women (King, 1989). Ten-year follow-up studies of patients with bulimia nervosa suggest that outcome is improved with intervention at an early stage, reinforcing the ideal of early diagnosis (Collings and King, 1994). Questionnaires such as the Eating Attitudes Test or EAT (Garner and Garfinkel, 1979) have good validity and contain useful probes, but if used on general at-risk populations may underestimate true morbidity, not least because of the tendency of anorexia nervosa sufferers to conceal their behaviour (Mann et al., 1983). Some studies have suggested that general practitioners are at least as sensitive as such screening questionnaires in detecting cases. Useful informal probes for abnormal eating behaviour in GP interviews might therefore be:

- how do you feel about your appearance?
- have you ever felt guilty about your weight?
- have you ever eaten something fattening to excess? If so, how often do you do this and, how do you feel afterwards? Do you ever make yourself sick?
- have you ever vomited/used purgatives/used diuretics/exercised a lot to try and control your weight?
- what weight would you like to be, ideally? (Compare to mean weight for age and height).
- (for women) have you stopped getting periods? (and for men) have you lost your sex drive?

The EAT has 40 questions on a self-rating 6 point Likert scale, with items like avoiding high carbohydrate food, feeling bloated after meals, feeling extremely guilty after eating, *weighing oneself several times a day, *being preoccupied with a desire to be thinner, *vomiting after eating, *taking laxatives. (Items marked * are the most significant. with a $p < 0.01$ on t-test.)

Physical examination may confirm the disorder in anorexia nervosa (low weight, bradycardia, peripheral cyanosis etc.) and contribute to the diagnosis in bulimia nervosa (parotid gland swelling, abrasions on the knuckles from inducing vomiting, poor dental enamel from gastric acid).

Treatable depression may affect some 10–15% of the population. Some 70% of cases will respond to pharmacological intervention with tricyclic or serotonin re-uptake inhibitors. Benefits in quality of life for the individual and for the family and society certainly make treatment worthwhile. In the elderly, depression has been linked to increased mortality from all causes of death, and in the elderly nearly all cases of depression are unrecognised and untreated. The depressed elderly commonly present (if they present at all) with physical symptoms rather than with psychological distress. Men have a different presentation pattern to women – with earlier recourse to alcohol, resulting dissocial behaviour and loss of job. To make the diagnosis in men requires a high index of suspicion for depressive illness and an increased willingness to treat, which in turn may yield considerable benefits of intervention by the general practitioner, as highlighted in the recent joint RCGP and RCPsych *Defeat Depression* campaign.

Useful probes to explore symptomatology would include a minimum set of questions about:

- crying or feeling like crying
- loss of interest in life and usual activities
- biological features (early morning wakening, diurnal mood variation, anorexia, weight loss and loss of sex drive)
- lack of things to look forward to
- a wish that life would end
- suicidal thoughts, impulses, fantasies and plans
- reliance on alcohol or drugs

Such probes betray a psychiatrist's model of depression. Many authors in general practice point to the very real difficulty in disentangling the presentation of anxiety from that of depression.

Psychiatrists, seeing the same patients, albeit it after referral and a time on a waiting list, tend to diagnose depression in the same patients earlier diagnosed by their GPs as anxiety disorder (Green and El-Hihi, 1990). This may reflect the worsening course of an illness where anxiety is often an initial presenting complaint.

Goldberg et al. (1988) have produced a validated short screening instrument for use in general medical settings, including general practice. The instrument has an anxiety scale and a depression scale.

ANXIETY SCALE

(Score one point for each positive response)

- have you felt keyed up, on edge?
- have you been worrying a lot?
- have you been irritable?
- have you had difficulty relaxing?

(if yes to two of the above go on to ask):

- have you been sleeping poorly?
- have you had headaches or neck-aches?
- have you had any of the following: trembling, tingling, dizzy spells, sweating, frequency, diarrhoea?
- have you been worried about your health?
- you had difficulty falling asleep?

DEPRESSION SCALE

(Score one point for each positive response)

- have you had low energy?
- have you had loss of interests?
- have you lost confidence in yourself?
- have you felt hopeless?

(If yes to any question go on to ask):

- have you had difficulty concentrating?
- have you lost weight (due to poor appetite)?
- have you been waking early?
- have you felt slowed up?
- have you tended to feel worse in the mornings?

(Interpretation – add the scores for the questions. People with anxiety scores over five and depression scores over two have *at least* a 50% chance of a clinically important disturbance).

Screening programmes for the elderly have been established in primary care, and since the prevalence of depression (about 10%) and dementia (about 5%) is relatively high in the over 65s, screening for these conditions is feasible. The presentation of depression in the aged is somewhat different to that of younger adults, consequently different screening instruments are required. The Evans Liverpool Depression Rating Scale (ELDRS) is a 15 point screening instrument validated against clinician and computer diagnoses of depression. It has proved useful in screening for depression amongst the elderly physically ill, and the residents of nursing homes.

ELDRS

Questions to ask the patient:

1. Have you been feeling sad or weepy recently?
2. What is your opinion of yourself compared with other people? Are you as good as other people your age, better, worse or the same?

If patient has a low opinion of him/herself ask:

3. Is there anything you feel guilty about or blame yourself for? What? (Only include unjustified or unreasonable guilt)
4. Do you worry about many things? Does this bother you?
5. Have you enough energy to do the things you want to do?
6. Did you get satisfaction or enjoyment from your life?
7. What do you think the future holds for you?

If patient is pessimistic about the future, ask:

8. Do you sometimes feel life is not worth living?
9. Have you ever felt that you would rather be dead?
10. Have you ever thought of harming yourself?

Questions to ask relatives or staff:

11. Is the patient socially isolating him/herself?
12. Does the patient complain of loneliness?
13. Has the patient been eating less well or lost any weight (in absence of known medical reason)?
14. Has the patient had trouble in sleeping: going to sleep, waking up early or taking medication for sleep?
15. Has the patient been irritable, bad tempered or snappish?

A score above 5 or 6 on the ELDRS gives the optimum sensitivity and specificity for depression screening purposes (Evans, 1993).

One of the hopes for screening programmes is that further deterioration can be reduced or that illness can be detected even before it becomes manifest. The latter pre-emptive or preventive strategy is not realistically available in psychiatry, although it is often hoped that early treatment may avoid later complication, for instance recognition and treatment of depression may save a marriage and avoid loss of employment, because colleagues may perceive illness as underperformance. Much effort has gone into epidemiological studies of depression to establish risk factors that might predict which people will develop the illness so that early intervention might be possible. In a longitudinal study of depression in the elderly, five risk factors reliably predicted the development of a first depressive illness three years later:

> *Bereavement of a close figure*
> *A lack of satisfaction with life*
> *Loneliness (but not living alone)*
> *Smoking*
> *and Female sex*

People who described their satisfaction with life as poor in response to the question "Taking everything into consideration . . . how would you describe your satisfaction with life in general at present: good, fair, or poor?" were at least three times as likely to develop depression three years later. Those who had lost a close figure through bereavement in the last six months were at least seven times more likely to develop depression three years later (Green et al., 1992). Whether psychological intervention with this at-risk group could have prevented later depressive illness is an interesting question, and one which might in the future be addressed through current screening activities in the elderly.

A shortened computer version of the Geriatric Mental State (Copeland et al., 1988) which probes for depression and dementia, and generates a computer validated diagnosis, has demonstrated good reliability and validity (Hoskins et al., 1994). The computer package used in general practice is called AGE-PC. Such a computerised test can be administered by nursing staff conducting simultaneous physical screening of the elderly.

Besides simple probes such as the above question about satisfaction with life, some attempts are made to assess quality of life. The concept of quality of life is not readily amenable to measurement, although there are scales which seek to do this (Neugarten et al., 1961). Quality of life is intrinsic to sophisticated cost-benefit analyses, and to the concept of mental health (Williams, 1990), although to date it remains an elusive and neglected construct.

Besides the AGE-PC package there are numerous single screening instruments for cognitive deficiencies such as in dementia. One of the tests found acceptable to primary care is the Mini-Mental State Examination (Folstein et al., 1975). Use of such instruments has been proposed should an acceptable treatment for Alzheimer's dementia be found (Wilcock et al., 1994). In the Wilcock et al. study, a cut-off score of below 23 was used as a guide to need for further detailed assessment.

Mini-Mental State Examination

Orientation:
What is the year? season? date? day? month?   Max. score 5
Where are we? Country? City? District? Street? House?   Max. score 5

Registration:
Name three objects (one second to say each)
Then ask the patient all 3 after you have said them.
                                    One point for each correct answer.

Attention and Concentration:
Serial Sevens (taking seven away from 100 and repeating the process):
Score one point for each correct answer. Stop after five answers.
Spell 'world' backwards.   Max. score 5

Recall:
Ask for the three objects repeated above. One point for each correct answer

Language:
Name a pencil and watch   (Two points)
Repeat the following : "No ifs, ands or buts".   (One point)
Follow a three-stage command: "Take a paper in your right hand,
fold it in half and put it on the floor"   (Three points)
Read and obey the following: 'Close your eyes'   (One point)
Write a sentence   (One point)
Copy design   (One point)

[Assess consciousness along a continuum: Alert/Drowsy/Stupor/Coma]

Audit Points

- *Which of these screening instruments could be used in your practice to identify psychological morbidity?*

- *What kind of protocol could be drawn up to manage patients who 'test positive' using such screening instruments?*

- *Many practices have adopted protocols for the treatment of anxiety or depression; many practices employ counsellors or psychotherapists; many practices work with psychologists or psychiatrists to produce psychological change in their patients.*

- *What outcomes do you expect when you treat or refer mental disorders? How can you quantify the changes you seek? If you see the desirable outcome in different terms to the screening instruments above, are there other validated instruments that might be useful to assess the impact of mental health interventions?*

References

Balint, M (1964) The Doctor, His Patient and the Illness. London, Pitman.

Collings, S, King, M. (1994) Ten-year follow-up of 50 patients with bulimia nervosa. British Journal of Psychiatry, 164, 80–87.

Copeland, J R M, Dewey M E, Henderson A S et al. (1988) The Geriatric Mental State (GMS) used in the community. Replication studies of the computerised diagnosis AGECAT. Psychological Medicine, 18, 219–223.

Copeland, J R M, Davidson, I A, Dewey, M E et al. (1992) Alzheimer's disease, other dementias, depression and pseudodementia: Prevalence, incidence and three-year outcome in Liverpool. British Journal of Psychiatry, 161, 230–239.

Evans, M. (1993) Development and validation of a brief screening scale for depression in the elderly physically ill. International Clinical Psychopharmacology, 8, 329–331.

Folstein M F, Folstein S E, McHugh, P R. (1975) Mini-mental state – a practical method for grading the cognition of patients for the clinician. Journal of Psychiatric Research, 12, 189–198.

Garner, D M, Garfinkel, P E. (1979) The Eating Attitudes Test: an index of the symptoms of anorexia nervosa. Psychological Medicine, 9, 273, 279.

Goldberg, D, Steele, J, Smith, C, Spivey L. (1980) Training family practice residents to recognise psychiatric disturbances. Final report, contract number ADMHA 278-78-003 (DB) Department of Psychiatry, Biometrics and Family Practice, Medical University of South Carolina.

Goldberg, D, Bridges, K, Duncan-Jones, P, Grayson, D. (1988) Detecting anxiety and depression in general medical settings. British Medical Journal, 297, 897–899.

Goldberg, D P, Huxley, P. (1992) Common Mental Disorders. A Bio-social Model. London, Tavistock/Routledge.

Green, B H, Copeland, J R M, Dewey M E et al. (1992) Risk factors for depression in elderly people: a prospective study. Acta Psychiatrica Scandinavica, 86, 213–217.

Green, B H, El-Hihi, M. (1990) Outpatient referrals of major depression to psychiatrists in central Liverpool. Psychiatric Bulletin, 14, 465–467.

Hoskins, A, Saunders, P A, Forrest, J M. (1994) A pilot study of a computerised assessment (AGE-PC) for the elderly in general practice. (In preparation)

Kessel, N, Walton, H. (1989) Alcoholism – a Reappraisal – its Causes, Problems and Treatment. 2nd edition, London, Penguin Books.

King, M B. (1989) Eating disorders in a general practice population: prevalence, characteristics and follow-up at 12–18 months. Psychological Medicine, suppl. 14, Cambridge University Press.

Mann, A H, Wakeling, A, Wood, K et al. (1983) Screening for abnormal eating attitudes and psychiatric morbidity in an unselected population of 15-year-old schoolgirls. Psychological Medicine, 13, 573–580.

Marks J N, Goldberg, D P, Hillier V F. (1979) Determinants of the ability of general practitioners to detect psychiatric illness. Psychological Medicine, 9, 337.

Mayfield, D, McLeod, G, Hall, P. (1974) The CAGE questionnaire: validation of a new alcoholism screening instrument. American Journal of Psychiatry, 131, 1121–1123.

Neugarten, B L, Havighurst R J, Tobin S S. (1961) The measurement of life satisfaction. Journal of Gerontology, 16, 134–143.

Pokorny, A D, Miller, B A, Kaplan, H B. (1972) The brief MAST: a shortened version of the Michigan alcoholism screening test. American Journal of Psychiatry, 129, 342–345.

Williams, A. (1990) Importance of quality of life. Measuring the benefits of medicines: the future agenda. (Edited by G Teeling Smith), London, Office of Health Economics.

Wilcock, G K, Ashworth, D L, Langfield Smith, P M. (1994) Detecting patients with Alzheimer's disease suitable for drug treatment: comparison of three methods of assessment. British Journal of General Practice, 44, 30–33.

Wilkins, R H (1974) The Hidden Alcoholic in General Practice. London, Elek.

Wooff K, Goldberg D P, Fryers, T. (1986). Patients in receipt of community psychiatric nursing in Salford 1976–1982. Psychological Medicine 16, 407.

Useful Addresses

Copies of the short and long versions of Goldberg's General Health Questionnaire, and many other mental health assessment instruments can be obtained from:

The NFER-NELSON Publishing Company Ltd.,
Darville House,
2, Oxford Road East,
Windsor, Berks, SL4 1DF.
Telephone: 0753-85961

Information about the AGE-PC assessment programme can be obtained through:

The Institute of Human Ageing,
The University of Liverpool,
P O Box 147,
Liverpool, L69 3BX.

Telephone: 051 794 5074

Mental Health Services

Dr Chris Dowrick

The preceding chapters have provided information about the prevalence of mental disorders in the community, and advice on how to diagnose or screen for such problems in patients presenting in general practice. At this stage, GPs may be forgiven for feeling somewhat overwhelmed by the extent and complexity of mental illness, and wondering whether they can possibly cope with the consequences of opening up such a Pandora's box!

There is a crucial distinction to be made between the ability to diagnose mental disorders, and the most appropriate methods of managing those disorders. GPs are and will remain the most common first professional port of call for patients with mental disorders (Goldberg and Huxley, 1992). We therefore have a professional obligation to recognise such problems, insofar as we are able to do so.

GPs are likely to wish to manage a proportion of mental health problems themselves, either through their own relationship with the patient (Balint, 1964) or through the effective use of antidepressant and anxiolytic medication. But it does not follow that we can or should take sole responsibility for providing all such care ourselves – this would place an impossible burden upon our own shoulders, and indeed deprive our patients of the opportunity to experience help from many other quarters.

GPs can therefore be seen as having two important roles to play in the management of patients with mental disorders. Firstly, as the *gatekeepers* to effective care; and secondly as *networkers*, as professionals with access to a wide range of suitable services.

This chapter is devoted to a description and discussion of the range of mental health services available to GPs and their patients. It is intended to provide GPs with a schema for considering possible avenues of help for their patients. Since not all services are standard across Britain, either in terms of quality or quantity, GPs will probably wish to customise the suggestions in this chapter in the light of their knowledge of local provision.

Mental health services, viewed from the perspective of general practice, may be divided into five categories, as shown below:

- Informal social networks
- The primary care team
- Self-help and voluntary groups
- Psychiatric services
- Social Service Departments

In addition to and overlapping with these categories, GPs also need to be aware of the implications of the new *community care* legislation for their patients with severe mental disorders: these are most likely to be patients with chronic schizophrenia, severe learning disabilities and dementia.

1. Informal social networks

- Family
- Friends
- Neighbours
- Social clubs
- Churches

The great majority of care for people suffering from mental disorders is undertaken by their families and neighbours. GPs should not use this as an excuse to neglect the appropriate use of or referral to other sources of help, nor ignore the immense burden that mental distress may impose on those close to the patient. It is nevertheless very important to be aware of the nature and extent of a patient's social network – including their involvement with churches, or with social clubs, and to consider the possibility of working with key members of that network to improve or maintain the patient's state of health.

In the management of depression for instance the presence or absence of a *confidante*, someone to whom the patient can turn to for support, tell all their troubles to, or trust with secrets, is a critical determinant of the speed with which they will recover from their illness. People with schizophrenia, on the other hand, are more likely to remain free of symptoms if they can live in an environment with *low expressed emotion*, that is to say where those around them are neither particularly critical of them nor demonstrably affectionate towards them.

2. The primary care team

- Counsellors
- Nurses
- Receptionists
- Educational materials

The person within the primary care team to whom the GP is most likely to turn for help is now the *practice counsellor*. The number of counsellors employed in general practice has increased enormously over the past decade (Pringle and Laverty, 1993). The public want access to counselling services within their neighbourhood, to provide support through major life events, and would like them located within primary care. In 1994 20% of all practices in the UK, and 50% of fundholding practices, employed a counsellor within their primary care team.

Counselling involves the 'skilled and principled use of relationships to help the client develop self-knowledge, emotional acceptance and growth, and personal resources' (Sheldon, 1992).

Who should be counselled?

Counselling is appropriate for people going through *transitions* – that is to say difficult life events such as bereavement, relationship problems – and who are becoming anxious or depressed as a result. It may also be helpful for people withdrawing from drugs or alcohol (Holden et al., 1989). It is less likely to benefit people with personality disorders or severe mental illness. Some GPs see counsellors as a useful dumping ground for their 'heartsink' patients. While a fresh approach may be helpful for some patients, that is generally unlikely to be an efficient use of counsellors' time.

Who should be counsellors?

Sibbald et al. (1993) found that counselling services were widespread in general practices in England and Wales, and that there are three main types of counsellors: community practice nurses, 'practice counsellors' and clinical psychologists. But they expressed concern that GPs were not always aware of the qualifications and experience of the counsellors they employed, that many counsellors appeared to lack relevant qualifications, and that they may be referred problems outside their knowledge. The British Association for Counselling have produced useful guidelines for the employment of counsellors in general practice (BAC, 1993).

Is counselling effective?

Corney (1990) has reviewed recent studies of counselling in primary care and found benefit in two-thirds of them. A recent study of counselling on Merseyside supports the contention that it is both more utilised and more effective for anxiety than for depressive symptoms (Dowrick and Fisher, in preparation). It seems likely that short-term focussed group work is more cost effective than long-term open-ended individual work, though it may also be more difficult to organise. Counselling may also have indirect benefits, in reducing costs of prescribing, hospital investigations and treatments (Sorby et al., 1991).

Many practices which do not (yet) employ counsellors will have access to counselling services in their locality. Information about these should be available through local libraries, Citizen's Advice Bureaux or Community Health Councils. GPs should be aware of the same caveats as for referring to in-house counselling.

Additionally, or alternatively, other members of the primary care team have important if less well defined roles to play in managing mental disorders. *Nursing colleagues* – particularly practice nurses – are able to detect mental health problems in the course of their clinical work, and may be offering an effective if often unrecognised counselling service to many patients. Several educational initiatives – such as the Take Care Programme currently being evaluated by the RCGP Research Unit in Manchester – are seeking to capitalise on this neglected resource. Similarly, *receptionists*, often caricatured as unhelpful dragons, in reality may possess and utilise high levels of counselling skills, of which GPs may be completely unaware.

Finally, there is now available a wide range of *educational materials*, such as booklets and tapes, to enable patients either to understand their problems more clearly or – particularly in the case of anxiety – to develop their own coping mechanisms more effectively (Donnan et al., 1990).

3. Self-help and voluntary groups

- Relate
- Cruse
- Alcoholics Anonymous
- MIND
- MENCAP etc.

There is a wide range of voluntary and non-statutory resources available in the community for patients with mental disorders, and these can be of enormous benefit to GPs and to patients.

Organisations such as Relate (previously the Marriage Guidance Council) and CRUSE exist to help people with specific problems arising from relationship difficulties or recent bereavements. Alcoholics Anonymous is well known, and most GPs will also be aware of Al-Anon, for the relatives of alcoholics, and of Gamblers Anonymous.

Patient advocacy groups may also be a significant source of help. MIND is a national charity working on behalf of people with mental health problems. It acts as a national educational and training organisation and a parliamentary pressure group. It is also committed to practical help at local level. In many parts of the country it organises drop-in centres, hotels and sheltered accomodation. MENCAP has a similar role on behalf of patients with learning difficulties.

The extent and quality of such resources will vary from one locality to another. Most GPs will have a mental note of some of the voluntary agencies available to their patients. It may be worth investing a little time – in the Citizens Advice Bureau or via local psychiatric or social service colleagues – in extending and systematising your knowledge of these services.

4. The psychiatric services

- Psychiatrists
- Community Psychiatric Nurses
- Clinical Psychologists
- Psychotherapists

The closure of mental hospitals and increasing emphasis on community care means that the old distinctions between primary and secondary care are rapidly becoming obsolete. Psychiatrists are increasingly working outside hospitals in community mental health teams. This trend has been broadly welcomed by general practitioners (Brown and Tower, 1990), but there is a need to clarify the roles and boundaries of the new relationship.

In terms of patient or diagnostic categories, there are clear spheres of interest and expertise at each end of the spectrum: transient social and psychological distress should remain in the domain of the primary care team, while acute psychotic episodes are best managed by psychiatrists. But there is a broad group in the middle – depression and chronic schizophrenia for instance – where either primary or secondary services could have a useful role. Co-operation between community mental health teams and primary care teams is likely to be both rational and cost-effective. General practitioners and psychiatrists need to come together to work out how best to manage this large 'middle ground'.

Creed and Marks (1989) have described the two main models of GP–psychiatrist cooperation. In the *shifted outpatient* model the psychiatrist sees outpatients in a primary care setting instead of a hospital. Patients prefer this to attending hospital, and it enables better access to GPs notes and better communication with GPs. In the *liaison-attachment* model the psychiatrist visits the primary care team on a regular basis, primarily for a liaison meeting and case discussion. The psychiatrist may also see a few patients either as formal referrals or with the general practitioner. This latter model appears to make more cost-effective use of psychiatric expertise: more patients are seen by psychiatrists – but more continue to be managed by the GP after one psychiatric consultation.

Community psychiatric nurses (CPNs) are set to play an increasingly prominent role in the management of mental disorders in the community. We have already noted their involvement in counselling services. Their main area of expertise, however, is in the maintenance and support of people with chronic mental disorders – primarily schizophrenia – in the community. GPs should be aware of them as an extremely valuable resource.

In some areas GPs have direct access to the services of CPNs, in others they need to approach them via local psychiatrists: it is therefore worth finding out what the arrangements are locally. Moreover, as general practice fundholding develops into the field of purchasing community nursing services, it is increasingly likely that CPNs will come to work more closely with, and indeed as part of, primary care teams.

GPs may also wish to make use of the scarce but significant services provided by *clinical psychologists* and *psychotherapists*, for help with patients whose problems appear too complex to be handled within the primary care team.

There are three broad approaches to be considered here:

- *Behavioural therapy* is most often carried out by clinical psychologists. It involves procedures such as relaxation training, modelling and systematic desensitisation. It is particularly useful for patients with specific identifiable problems, such as phobias, obsessional disorders, chronic pain or poor social skills.

- *Psychodynamic therapy* is the domain of psychotherapists. It analyses problems as stemming largely from unresolved conflicts in early childhood, and helps the patient to recognise and come to terms with the origins of these problems. It is most likely to be useful with patients who can understand their problems in psychological terms, can communicate verbally, and can tolerate pain and distress in the context of a therapeutic relationship.

- An important recent development is *cognitive-behavioural therapy*, which concentrates on patients' thoughts. It works from the premise that patients can be responsible for their actions, and that they can modify their patterns of thinking from negative to positive 'schema' (Blackburn and Davidson, 1990). *Cognitive analytical therapy* (CAT) is a highly effective synthesis of cognitive and psychodynamic approaches (Ryle, 1991).

5. Social services departments

- People
  Social Workers
  Care Assistants
- Places
  Hostels
  Group Homes
  Day Centres

As we have already seen in the section on Mental Health legislation, social workers have statutory involvement in the management of extreme mental disorders through compulsory admissions ('Sections') to psychiatric hospitals. Unfortunately, such stressful and explosive encounters may be the only time that GPs come into contact with social work colleagues, and they are hardly the most auspicious circumstances for developing a useful knowledge of each other's roles.

In fact many social workers have considerable training and expertise in mental health work (Goldberg and Huxley, 1992, Ch. 10). The Edinburgh depression study (Scott and Freeman, 1992) found that the problem solving approach adopted by social workers produced more rapid relief from depression than cognitive therapy, antidepressants prescribed by a psychiatrist or GP's normal management.

Social workers also have access to a wide variety of resources, such as day centres, hostels and group homes, which may be of considerable benefit to patients with more chronic mental health problems. And they are of central importance in the new arrangements for community care.

Community care

During the 1980s there was considerable concern about two main groups of mentally disordered patients: those with chronic schizophrenia, and elderly patients with dementia. Changes in the community care legislation introduced in April 1993 have been designed to improve the situation of these patients, and GPs have an important role to play.

Community care for schizophrenic patients has often proved inadequate; indeed services appeared to deteriorate with the rapid closure of many large mental institutions during the 1980s (Murphy, 1992). Many discharged patients continue to be disturbed by psychotic experiences, have poor or no accomodation, receive little social support and have no prospect of employment. Those patients living with their families can cause enormous emotional strain.

Many elderly patients with dementia have been inadequately supported at home or else placed inappropriately in residential or nursing homes. Throughout the 1980s there was a perverse incentive, based on the availability of financial assistance from the Department of Social Security, towards institutional rather than community care for frail elderly people.

The Health and Community Care Act, often referred to as 'Caring for People' has been designed to redress these problems. It invests power in Social Service Departments to organise appropriate community-based care for patients with severe mental and physical health problems. This is leading to a significant transfer of resources from institutional to community-based services over a five-year period. As long as the total budget is not reduced, it should allow for a more effective range of community provision for these patients. The two main ingredients of the new approach are *care assessment*, when patients are offered a comprehensive review of their problems and the services they may need, and *care management*, when a planned package of care is set up for patients who are particularly at risk.

These developments overlap with changes already taking place in the way psychiatric teams organise the care of their patients when in the community rather than in hospital. They allocate one member of the team – psychiatrist, social worker or community psychiatric nurse – to become the *keyworker*. The keyworker is the contact point between the patient and the psychiatric services. He or she has the responsibility to ensure that the patient's needs are fully assessed and that a realistic care plan is drawn up.

The Secretary of State for Health is, at the time of writing, considering extending this system by requiring hospitals to draw up registers of severely mentally ill patients who have been discharged into the community. It is not clear whether this proposal is designed primarily for the benefit of the patients themselves, or as a reaction to publicity surrounding the discharge of the small numbers of mentally ill patients who commit serious crimes.

Community psychiatric nurses and social workers are likely to take the major responsibility for care assessment and management. GPs will certainly have a role in informing the process of assessment of their patients. Those with a greater interest may also wish to make use of recent educational initiatives, such as the work of Tony Kendrick at St George's Hospital, London, designed to provide regular practice-based reviews of patients with chronic mental illness. Fundholding GPs who are expanding their work with community nursing teams may also wish to consider taking on the care management budgets for their own patients (Dowrick, 1992).

- Shift of resources from institutional to community care
- Care assessment
- Care management
- Possible roles for GPs:
    informing assessments
    reviews of long term mentally ill patients
    fundholding and care management

CASE VIGNETTES:

1. A 51-year old man comes to see you complaining of headaches and general malaise. He has not consulted you or your partners for over a year. You discover that he has been 'away' in prison for the past 8 months, following a conviction for fraud. You also discover that as a consequence of this, he has been sacked from his job and his marriage has ended. Not surprisingly, he is severely depressed – though not suicidal – and has been drinking heavily since his release from prison 2 weeks ago.

    What resources, apart from a psychiatric opinion or a course of antidepressants, might be helpful for this man?

2. A 20-year old woman comes for a repeat of the pill, and for advice about a flare-up of a patch of eczema on her right wrist. On enquiry into the causes of the exacerbation for her eczema, you find out that she is mildly depressed. She rarely goes out of the house. She is unemployed and is living alone with her 3-year-old son. Her extended family live nearby but she sees little of them. She may have a boyfriend – hence the prescription for the pill – but as far as you can tell he does not figure significantly in her life.

    Do you consider that this patient's social isolation and mild depression are problems a GP should get involved with? If so, who in the primary care team or beyond, could help?

3. A 30-year-old man with chronic schizophrenia has come to see you for a repeat prescription of his antipsychotic medication. His mental state is stable, and gives you no particular cause for concern. You take a few minutes to enquire into his current lifestyle and discover that he is living with his mother aged 69, and appears to do very little with himself apart from going shopping and the occasional unsuccessful flutter on the horses.

    What services might you wish to offer him, with the intention of enriching his life, or giving some support to his mother?

Audit Points

- *How much do you already know about the local availability of mental health services for your patients? Where do you store this information? In your head, or on a card index/computer index/practice leaflet? How can you find out about hitherto unexplored resources?*

- *What use do you make of these resources? You might wish to undertake a retrospective or prospective audit of your referral patterns for mental health problems, using the five categories outlined in this chapter. How do your patterns compare with your partners? How and why might you wish to modify them?*

USEFUL ADDRESSES

British Association of Counselling: 1 Regent Place, Rugby, CV21 2PJ, Tel: 0778 550899

MIND, Granta House, 15–19 Broadway, London, E15 4BQ, Tel: 081 519 2122

MENCAP, 123 Golden Lane, London, EC1Y 0RT, Tel: 071 454 0454

REFERENCES

Balint, M. (1964) The Doctor, His Patient and the Illness. London, Pitman.

Blackburn I, Davidson K. (1990) Cognitive Therapy for Depression and Anxiety. Oxford, Blackwell.

British Association of Counsellors. (1993) Guidelines for the Employment of Counsellors in General Practice. Rugby, BAC.

Brown M, Tower EC. (1990) Psychiatrists in general practice: would general practitioners welcome them? British Journal of General Practice, 40, 369–371.

Corney R. (1990) Counselling in general practice: does it work? Journal of the Royal Society of Medicine, 83, 253–257.

Creed F, Marks B. (1989) Liaison psychiatry in general practice: a comparison of the liaison attachment scheme and the shifted outpatient clinic models. Journal of the Royal College of General Practitioners, 39, 514–517.

Donnan P, Hutchinson A, Paxton R, et al. (1990) Self-help materials for anxiety: a randomised controlled trial in general practice. British Journal of General Practice, 40, 498–501.

Dowrick C. (1992) Who will be 'Caring for people'? British Journal of General Practice, 42, 2–3.

Goldberg D, Huxley P. (1992) Common Mental Disorders – a Biosocial Model. London, Routledge.

Holden J M, Sagovsky R, Cox J L. (1989) Counselling in a general practice setting: controlled study of health visitor intervention in treatment of postnatal depression. British Medical Journal, 298, 223–226.

Murphy E. (1992) After the Asylums. London, Faber.

Pringle M, Laverty J. A counsellor in every practice? British Medical Journal, 306, 2–3.

Ryle A. (1991) Cognitive Analytic Therapy: Active Participation in Change. Chichester, John Wiley and Sons.

Scott A I, Freeman C P. (1992) The Edinburgh primary care depression study: treatment outcome, patient satisfaction, and cost after 16 weeks. British Medical Journal, 304, 883–887.

Sheldon M (ed). (1992) Counselling in General Practice. London, RCGP.

Sibbald B, Addington-Hall J, Brenneman D, Freeling P. (1993) Counsellors in English and Welsh general practices: their nature and distribution. Briitish Medical Journal, 306, 29–33.

Sorby N G D, Reavley W, Huber J W. (1991) Self-help programme for anxiety in general practice: controlled trial of an anxiety management booklet. Briitish Journal of General Practice, 41, 417–420.

Glossary

Affect A person's affect is their immediate emotional state which the person can recognise subjectively and which can also be recognised objectively by others. A person's mood is their predominant current affect.

Agnosia An inability to organise sensory information so as to recognise objects (e.g. visual agnosia) or sometimes even parts of the body (e.g. hemisomatoagnosia).

Akathisia An inner feeling of excessive restlessness which provokes the sufferer to fidget in their seat or pace about.

Anxiety Anxiety is provoked by fear or apprehension and also results from a tension caused by conflicting ideas or motivations. Anxiety manifests through mental and somatic symptoms such as palpitations, dizziness, hyperventilation, and faintness.

Compulsion The behavioural component of an obsession. The individual feels compelled to repeat a behaviour which has no immediate benefit beyond reducing the anxiety associated with the obsessional idea. For instance for a person obsessed by the idea that they are dirty, repeated ritual handwashing may serve to reduce anxiety.

Confabulation Changing, loosely held and false memories created to fill in organically-derived amnesia

Deja vu An abnormal experience where an individual feels that a particular or unique event has happened before in exactly the same way.

Delirium An acute organic brain syndrome secondary to physical causes in which consciousness is affected and disorientation results often associated with illusions, visual hallucinations and persecutory ideation.

Delusion An incorrect belief which is out of keeping with the person's cultural context, intelligence and social background and which is held with unshakeable conviction.

Delusional mood	Also known as *Wahnstimmung*, a feeling that something unusual is about to happen of special significance for that person.
Delusional perception	A normal perception which has become highly invested with significance and which has become incorporated into a delusional system, e.g. 'when I saw the traffic lights turn red I knew that the dog I was walking was a Nazi and a lesbian Nazi at that'.
Dementia	A chronic organic mental illness which produces a global deterioration in cognitive abilities and which usually runs a deteriorating course.
Depersonalisation	An experience where the self is felt to be unreal, detached from reality or different in some way. Depersonalisation can be triggered by tiredness, dissociative episodes or partial epileptic seizures.
Depression	An affective disorder characterised by a profound and persistent sadness.
Derealisation	An experience where the person perceives the world around them to be unreal. The experience is linked to depersonalisation.
Echolalia	A speech disorder in which the person inappropriately and automatically repeats the last words he or she has heard. Palilalia is a form of echolalia in which the last syllable heard is repeated endlessly.
Echopraxia	A movement disorder in which the person automatically and inappropriately imitates or mirrors the movements of another.
First rank symptoms	Schneider classified the most characteristic symptoms of schizophrenia as first-rank features of schizophrenia. These included third person auditory hallucinations, thought echo, thought interference (insertion, withdrawal, and broadcasting), delusional perception and passivity phenomena.
Flight of ideas	In mania and hypomania thoughts become pressured and ideas may race from topic to topic, guided sometimes only by rhymes or puns. Ideas are associated, however, unlike thought disorder.
Frontal lobe syndrome	This follows frontal lobe damage or may be consequent upon a lesion such as a tumour or infarction. There is a lack of judgement, a coarsening of personality, disinhibition, pressure of speech, lack of planning ability, and sometimes apathy. Perseveration and a return of the grasp reflex may occur.

PART 1: PRINCIPLES

Hallucination	An abnormal sensory experience that arises in the absence of a direct external stimulus, and which has the qualities of a normal percept and is experienced as real and usually in external space. Hallucinations may occur in any sensory modality.
Hypomania	An affective disorder characterised by elation, overactivity, and insomnia.
Illusion	An abnormal perception caused by a sensory misinterpretation of an actual stimulus, sometimes precipitated by strong emotion, e.g. fear provoking a person to imagine they have seen an intruder in the shadows.
Insight	In psychotic mental disorders and organic brain syndromes a patient's insight into whether or not they are ill and therefore requiring treatment may be affected. In depression a person may lack insight into their best qualities and in mania a person may overestimate their wealth and abilities.
Jamais vu	An abnormal experience where an individual feels that a routine or familiar event has never happened before. (See deja vu).
Made experiences	See 'Passivity phenomena'.
Mania	An affective disorder characterised by intense euphoria, overactivity and loss of insight.
Neologism	A novel word often invented and used in schizophrenic thought disorder.
Obsession	An unpleasant or nonsensical thought which intrudes into a person's mind, despite a degree of resistance by the person who recognises the thought as pointless or senseless, but nevertheless a product of their own mind. Obsessions may be accompanied by compulsive behaviours which serve to reduce the associated anxiety.
Parietal lobe signs	Parietal lobe signs include various agnosias (such as visual agnosias, sensory neglect, and tactile agnosias), dyspraxias (such as dressing dyspraxia), body image disturbance, and hemipareses or hemiplegias.

Passivity phenomena — In these phenomena the individual feels that some aspect of themselves is under the external control of another or others. These may therefore include 'made acts and impulses' where the individual feels they are being made to do something by another, 'made movements' where their arms or legs feel as if they are moving under another's control, 'made emotions' where they are experiencing someone else's emotions, and 'made thoughts' which are categorised elsewhere as thought insertion and withdrawal.

Perseveration — Describes an inappropriate repetition of some behaviour or thought or speech. Echolalia is an example of perseverative speech. Talking exclusively on one subject might be described as perseveration on a theme. Perseveration of thought indicates an inability to switch ideas, so that in an interview a patient may continue to give the same responses to later questions as he did to earlier ones. Perseveration is sometimes a feature of frontal lobe lesions.

Schizophasia — A severe form of thought disorder.

Tardive dyskinesia — An abnormal involuntary movement disorder which may manifest as lip-smacking bucco-lingual movements or grimacing, truncal movements or athetoid limb movements.

Thought blocking — The unpleasant experience of having one's train of thought curtailed absolutely, often more a sign than a symptom.

Thought broadcasting — The experience that one's thoughts are being transmitted from one's mind and broadcast to everyone.

Thought disorder — A disorder of the form of thought, where associations between ideas are lost or loosened.

Thought echo — Where thoughts are heard as if spoken aloud, when there is some delay these are known as *echo de la pensée* and when heard simultaneously, *Gedankenlautwerden*.

Thought insertion — The experience of alien thoughts being inserted into the mind.

Thought withdrawal — The experience of thoughts being removed or extracted from one's mind.

Word salad — A severe form of thought disorder.